Tell Me What to Eat to Help Prevent Colon Cancer

Nutrition You Can Live With

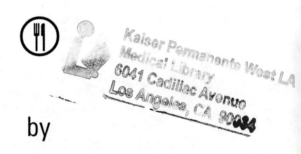
by

Elaine Magee, MPH, RD

New Page Books
A division of The Career Press, Inc.
Franklin Lakes, NJ

TELL ME WHAT TO EAT TO HELP PREVENT COLON CANCER
Edited by Robert M. Brink
Typeset by John J. O'Sullivan
Cover design by Lu Rossman
Printed in the U.S.A. by Book-mart Press

To order this title, please call toll-free 1-800-CAREER-1 (NJ and Canada: 201-848-0310) to order using VISA or MasterCard, or for further information on books from Career Press.

The Career Press, Inc., 3 Tice Road, PO Box 687,
Franklin Lakes, NJ 07417
www.newpagebooks.com
www.careerpress.com

Library of Congress Cataloging-in-Publication Data
Magee, Elaine.
  Tell me what to eat to prevent colon cancer : nutrition you can
  Live with / by Elaine Magee.
    p.cm. – (Tell me what to eat)
  Includes index.
  ISBN 1- 56414-514 X (pbk.)
    1. Colon (Anatomy)—Cancer—Prevention—Popular works. 2.
  Colon (Anatomy)—Cancer—Diet therapy—Popular works. I.
  Title. II. Series.

RC280.C6 M325 2001
616.99'434705—dc21   00-046539

Contents

Introduction 5

Chapter 1:
Everything You Ever Wanted to Ask Your Doctor
   About Colon Cancer 7

Chapter 2:
The Diet and Colon Cancer Connection 19

Chapter 3:
Everything You Ever Wanted to Ask Your Dietitian
   About Colon Cancer 29

Chapter 4:
10 Food Steps to Freedom 39

Chapter 5:
Focus on Health...Not Pounds 89

Chapter 6:
Recipes You Cannot Live Without 101

Chapter 7:
Navigating the Supermarket 122

Chapter 8:
Restaurant Rules 142

Index 157

Introduction

'm turning 39 in a month and let me tell you, after research-
ing and writing this book, I'm volunteering for a colonoscopy
by my 40th birthday. I'm going to have one done at 50, 60,
and hopefully, I'll be around to have it repeated at 70 too. It's
about a two-day time investment and from what I've heard, the
day before the procedure is the worst. The day is apparently split
between drinking a horrible tasting solution and running to the
bathroom. According to my experienced friends, it's all down hill
from there.

After this two-day ordeal you are well screened for colon cancer, any polyps found have been removed, and the procedure is
good for 10 years. I don't know about you, but I feel this is one of
the best medical deals going. If there were something similar for
ovarian cancer I'd be signing up for that too.

Here's why you should care...

- Colon cancer is the second deadliest cancer in the
  United States.

- The American Cancer Society estimates there are over 130,000 new cases of colorectal cancer each year, with about 55,000 deaths from it each year.
- If you don't smoke, and your breast or prostate stay cancer-free, the biggest cancer risks are your colon and rectum.

The good news

Nine of 10 deaths associated with colon cancer can be avoided. The key is finding and removing pre-malignant polyp growths called adenomas (they usually take a decade to become cancerous growths). The American Institute of Cancer Research estimates that as many as 75 percent of colon cancer cases are preventable by diet.

There are three steps to preventing colon cancer:

1. Screening.
2. Minimizing exposure to carcinogens.
3. Maximizing exposure to substances that help protect the body against these carcinogens.

A healthy diet is a large part of what Chapters 2 and 3 (as well as the rest of this book) are all about. You will read about the common screening tests for colon cancer and how to minimize exposure to carcinogens in Chapter 1.

The thought of any type of cancer is very real and very scary for most of us. This book is about turning that fear into something positive and productive. I personally feel better if I keep current with all my different screenings, and if I take common-sense steps with diet and lifestyle to reduce my risk of cancer. Beyond that, it's out of my hands.

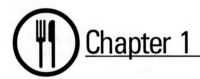 Chapter 1

Everything You Ever Wanted to Ask Your Doctor About Colon Cancer

Q **What exactly is a "colon" and what's this word I keep hearing...colorectal?**

First, let me explain what the large intestine is and what it does. Then you'll understand what the colon is. After food travels through the stomach and small intestine (where food is digested and calories and nutrients are absorbed), any material left over passes into the large intestine, which has two parts—the colon and the rectum. The colon is the upper five or six feet of the large intestine and rectum is the lower five or six inches (the part that reaches the anus, where waste exits the body).

Because the tissues and cancer tumors that appear in the colon and rectum are so similar, the names for cancers of the colon and rectum are often combined as "colorectal cancer."

Q **What is colon cancer?**

Colon cancer is when cells in the colon grow out of control, forming a small group of abnormal cells. These cells grow into a lump called a polyp, which is a small, non-cancerous tumor that may turn into cancer.

Q **What causes colon cancer?**
Unfortunately we do not yet know the exact causes of colon cancer. What we do know is that both inherited and environmental factors may lead to colon cancer.

One proposed hypothesis is that bile acids promote the development of colon cancer, so scientists have been looking to foods and medications (such as hormone therapy) that reduce the production of these bile acids.

Q **How does it spread to other organs in the body?**
You might hear the word "metastasis" or "metastasized" in reference to colon cancer. Metastasis is when cancer cells have spread to other parts of the body. How does this happen? First the colorectal tumors develop inside the colon or rectum. Then, after a certain point in the life of the tumor, some of the cells break away from the tumor and enter the bloodstream or lymph system, possibly forming new tumors in other parts of the body.

Q **What's a polyp, and why are they important?**
Most colorectal cancers begin as non-cancerous overgrowths of cells called polyps. You might also come across the more medical term "adenomatous polyps" and the definition: visible protrusions that develop on the mucosal surface of the colon or rectum.

Polyps can bleed or interfere with the large intestine's doing its job. Most can be removed. But they may become cancerous if they aren't removed in time.

Polyps are found in the colons of about 30 percent of people by age 50. By age 70, the number jumps to 50 percent. However, less than 1 percent of these lesions ever become cancerous. Experts estimate that it takes an average of 10 years for a polyp to become malignant (cancerous). Experts don't know why some polyps eventually become cancerous, but think it may have to do with genetic changes in colon cells over long periods of time.

When the doctors look at a polyp they consider its size, the organization of the cells within it, and the look of the cells themselves. Flat, long, or stalk-shaped cells may be cancerous.

Q Who's at risk?
Age: Anyone at any age can get colon cancer. People age 50 and older are most likely to get this disease. Why? Because as we age, our cells don't repair themselves as well, and genetic changes within the colon tissue predispose cells to grow out of normal control.

Gender: Both men and women get colon cancer, but men are slightly more likely to develop colorectal cancer. They are also more likely to die from it.

Ethnicity: In the United States, rates are higher among African-Americans, Japanese-Americans, and non-Hispanic whites than among other ethnic groups.

Worldwide: Colorectal cancer rates are highest in North America, northern and western Europe, and Australia, and are lowest in Asia and Africa. One of the biggest clues that diet and lifestyle are related to colon cancer risk comes from looking at immigrants. People who come from a country with a low incidence of colon cancer (like Japan), to a country with a higher incidence of colon cancer (like the U.S.), end up mimicking these higher cancer rates within the first and second generations. If colon cancer were entirely genetic, then we wouldn't see a shift in the risk.

People who have any of the following are considered to be at higher risk for colon cancer:

- A parent, sibling, or child with colon cancer or polyps has two to four times the risk (according to studies by Columbia University and Memorial Sloan-Kettering).
- A family history of breast, ovarian, uterine, stomach or liver cancer also may increase your likelihood, but exactly how much is not yet known.
- A personal history of polyps can triple your risk.
- Your risk of getting this cancer also increases by 30 percent if you've had chronic inflammatory conditions, such as ulcerative colitis or Crohn's disease, for eight years or more.

According to the *Harvard Health Letter,* people with at least one first-degree relative (mother, father, child, or sibling) who has had colorectal and ovarian or endometrial cancers probably have a genetic predisposition to the disease. They should undergo screening at a younger age and possibly more frequently than the general population (Nov. 1, 1998 vol. 24).

People who smoke or are sedentary (having a low physical activity level) have a higher risk for colorectal cancer. For information on the food and diet related risk factors for colorectal cancer, see Chapter 3.

Adults who do not have genetic or other specific symptoms or factors putting them at high risk, are automatically considered at average risk for colon cancer when they reach age 50. The chance of an average-risk patient developing invasive colorectal cancer is one in 19.

Q **What percentage of colon cancer can be attributed to heredity/genetics?**
This answer depends on whom you ask. Of the 130,000 cases of colon cancer diagnosed each year, 50 to 85 percent have no major genetic component, according to Johns Hopkins University researcher Steven Laken. Other researchers estimate that 5 to 10 percent of all colon cancer is considered hereditary. I find this interesting because about the same percentage of breast cancer is genetically related.

Q **What can I do if I have colon cancer in my family?**
There are many things you can do to find out if you have a genetic predisposition to colon cancer. In the past few years, genetic tests have become available for two forms of inherited colorectal cancer:

- Familial Adenomatous Polyposis (FAP), a rare type of colon cancer that strikes people under the age of 40. This test is now commercially available.
- Hereditary NonPolyposis Colorectal Cancer (HNPCC, also called Lynch syndrome), the most common inherited form, often diagnosed by age 45 or 50. Families with this type of colon cancer also usually have family members with ovarian, endometrial, or other

cancers. This test is, at the time of publication, still considered experimental and offered only through certain research institutions.

Note: Genetic screening for FAP or HNPCC should only be done along with genetic counseling and the tests only indicate whether someone has a higher than average risk of getting the disease.

The bottom line is that you have to get yourself in for screening early enough and then keep up the schedule (every 10 years for a colonoscopy). If you have a genetic tendency to colon cancer you should still follow the lifestyle and diet suggestions to help prevent colon cancer. These steps may postpone the development of colon cancer.

Q **What are the signs and symptoms of colon cancer I should be looking for?**

The early stages of colon cancer are usually without symptoms. The following are warning signs of an intestinal tumor, but can also be caused by other factors—from the flu to stress. If any of the following symptoms persist, it's important to see a doctor immediately to determine the cause.

- A prolonged change in bowel habits (diarrhea or constipation).
- A constant feeling of having to go to the bathroom (or a feeling that the bowel hasn't emptied completely).
- Rectal bleeding or blood in the stool (either bright red or very dark in color).
- Stomach discomfort (cramps, bloating, or fullness).
- Frequent gas pains.
- Decreased appetite and/or weight loss with no known reason.
- Abnormal weakness and fatigue.
- Stools that are narrower than usual.
- Vomiting.
- Unexplained anemia (low levels of iron in the blood).

- Jaundice (yellow-green discoloration of the skin and white part of the eyes).

These symptoms may be caused by colorectal cancer or by other conditions. It is important to check with your doctor.

Q **Should I be screened for colon cancer? At what age?**
Yes, and it depends. Stating the obvious, the earlier you catch colon cancer, the better. A recent expert panel (appointed by the Agency for Health Care Policy and Research) determined about 18,000 more lives could be saved each year if more people were simply screened by the age of 50.

Routine screening helps to detect cancer tumors in their earliest, most treatable stages. This can be very effective. If the cancer is detected early, 90 percent of the cases can be cured. Unfortunately, only 40 percent of colon cancer cases are caught early. According to the Harvard Health Letter, once the cancer spreads to the lymph nodes, the five-year survival rate drops to 50 percent. If the disease has spread to the liver, the survival rate plummets to less than 3 percent (Nov. 1, 1998 vol. 24).

Here are some of the screening options available:

Fecal Occult Blood Testing (FOBT)

These laboratory kits cost about $8 and they are the most common colon cancer screening tests, although their effectiveness is being questioned. This test involves taking samples from two different parts of your stool, for three days, and spreading the samples on the testing paper. A recent study found a 33 percent reduction in death (in average-risk people) from colorectal cancer in the group having an annual FOBT test. Some of this reduction in risk could be due to colonoscopies that were performed due to false positive FOBT results. If you are opting for an FOBT as part of your annual physical exam, there are a few things you might want to know:

- Of all the different FOBT tests available, HemeSelect (an immunochemical test) has been shown to perform better than the others.

- The test is more accurate (avoiding false-negative and false-positive test results) when you abstain from taking aspirin and eating certain foods (red meat, some raw fruits and vegetables, and vitamin C supplements). Be sure to ask your doctor if there are any food guidelines he/she wants you to follow before taking the samples.
- It can still miss a cancer that wasn't bleeding at the time or it can pick up bleeding for which no source can be found.

Flexible sigmoidoscopy

This test involves a flexible fiber-optic probe (sigmoidoscope) that views the lining of the rectum and the last two feet of colon in search for polyps. This test usually doesn't require sedation and costs about $135. The downside to this is that the area of the colon examined by the scope typically contains only half of the possible polyps. Some physicians liken it to only checking one breast during a mammography. The other downside is that if a polyp is found, you will have to come back at another time for a follow-up colonoscopy test. This will view the entire colon with a longer endoscope and remove the polyps seen during the previous sigmoidoscopy. This test is not recommended for hereditary nonpolyposis colon cancer screening because about two thirds of the lesions in these cases develop in the upper portion of the colon, not reached by the sigmoidoscope.

Colonoscopy

This is a more involved test, recommended for high-risk people or when the other tests (FOBT, sigmoidoscopy, or barium enema) results are positive. This test will view the colon, biopsy necessary areas, and remove any pre-cancerous or early-stage cancerous polyps in one step.

The downside to this procedure:
- The test is performed in a hospital or certified endoscopy unit and can cost around $500 plus hospital charges.

Screening recommendations

Who	Recommendation
The U.S. Preventive Services Task Force	People 50 years and older without symptoms should be screened annually with FOBT and Sigmoidoscopy at unspecified intervals. High-risk patients should be referred to a subspecialist.
The World Health Organization	Sigmoidoscopy at age 10 to 12 for patients with familial adenomatous polyposis.
National Cancer Institute and American Cancer Society	Annual digital rectal examination for all adults beginning at age 40 and two tests for average-risk persons beginning at age 50; annual FOBT (with rehydration) and flexible sigmoidoscopy every 3 to 5 years. Colonoscopy is recommended for high-risk individuals.
American College of Obstetricians and Gynecologists	FOBT for all women 40 and older as part of their annual examination.
American College of Physicians	Suggest offering flexible sigmoidoscopy, colonoscopy, or barium enema to patients aged 50 to 70, depending on resources and preferences, and repeating tests every 10 years. FOBT should be offered starting at age 40 to patients at high risk.
American College of Radiology	Screening with barium enema every 3 to 5 years.

- Patients are usually asked to eat a low-residue or clear liquid diet for 24 hours before the procedure. They are also sedated during the procedure.

- There is a one-in-500 risk of perforation of the colon during the procedure.
- Aspirin and nonsteroidal anti-inflammatory drugs should be discontinued one week before, due to the possibility of bleeding during the procedure.
- Abdominal cramping can occur during and after the procedure.
- Colonoscopy isn't recommended for those with fulminant colitis, recent colectomy, known or suspected perforation, unstable cardiorespiratory condition, or coagulopathy.

Sigmoidoscopy and colonoscopy; not as bad as they sound

I can think of a lot more enjoyable things to do than to have a barium enema followed by a flexible sigmoidoscope or colonoscope traveling through my colon. But these procedures can save your life by detecting and removing polyps before they become cancerous, or by finding a cancerous tumor while it is still treatable. I guess you could say the first sigmoidoscopy or colonoscopy is probably going to be your worst. Once you've gone through the procedure you realize it isn't as bad as it sounds. Many people report that they were not significantly uncomfortable during or after the test and it was not as bad as they expected.

(Air-contrast) barium enema

The test looks at the entire colon and costs about $200. During this test, air and barium are placed in the colon through the rectum and an X-ray of the entire colon is taken. This test alone isn't as effective or sensitive as the scope tests are. Sometimes false positive results occur (leading to unnecessary colonoscopies). Large polyps and tumors are identified with this test but the smaller cancers and precancerous lesions may go unnoticed.

Digital (finger) rectal examination

This is a simple, safe, and inexpensive test often performed by your doctor during an annual exam. The only trouble is, it only works if the polyps develop within the seven-centimeter reach of the examining finger.

•••

Many physicians and researchers choose to follow the American Cancer Society recommendation for annual FOBT, but they limit the flexible sigmoidoscopy for average-risk persons to every five years. For high-risk patients, they perform interval colonoscopy every three to five years, starting at an age 10 to 15 years younger than the age of the youngest affected relative. For example, if your father developed colorectal cancer at age 53, interval colonoscopy would begin for you at age 38 to 43.

Scientists are developing new noninvasive imaging tests that may, in the next few years, replace the aforementioned endoscopic examinations. So stay tuned.

Q **If I get a colonoscopy, will the entire colon be screened?** For the most part, but the scope may not reach the cecum—the pouch of tissue that joins the large and small intestines. About 20 percent of colon cancers occur in this portion of the colon.

Q **What is the most common treatment for colorectal cancer?** Surgically removing the tumor is the most common treatment. Usually the surgeon removes the tumor along with part of the healthy colon or rectum and nearby lymph nodes. In most cases, the doctor is able to reconnect the healthy portions of the colon or rectum.

Other treatments, including chemotherapy, radiation therapy, and immunotherapy may be used, depending on the situation.

Q **What is a colostomy?** If the surgeon cannot reconnect the healthy portions of the colon during surgery, a temporary or permanent colostomy (a surgical opening through the wall of the abdomen into the colon which provides a new path for food waste to leave the body), usually follows. The patient wears a special bag to collect the waste. Sometimes patients need a temporary colostomy just long enough to help the colon heal after surgery. Maybe 5 percent of colorectal cancer patients end up needing a permanent colostomy.

Q **What else can I do to help prevent colon cancer?**
Besides the genetic link, other risks that have been suggested for colon cancer include ulcerative colitis and Crohn's disease, a history of smoking, excessive alcohol use, being overweight, a sedentary lifestyle, and a diet low in fruits, vegetables, and dietary fiber.

Minimize exposure to carcinogens

Not smoking and avoiding people when they smoke is a big step in the right direction. Avoiding carcinogenic chemicals and radiation will also help.

Hormone Replacement Therapy

Estrogen replacement therapy (and estrogen in combination with progestin) is suggested to substantially decrease colon cancer risk in postmenopausal women. Although this conclusion is still controversial, researchers suspect that the hormone estrogen exerts a protective effect. This has not been proven and experts don't recommend using it exclusively for colon protection. The suspected connection is that hormone therapy reduces the production of bile acids.

Aspirin

If you are at risk for a heart attack, you might already be taking an aspirin a day. So you might be encouraged to note that plain old aspirin has been shown to prevent some colorectal polyps from forming (including in people who have already had polyps removed). Additionally, it causes the regression of small adenomas in people with familial adenomatous polyposis. Recent data (from the Nurse's Health Study) showed that taking four to six regular-strength tablets per week, for at least 10 years, reduced the risk of colorectal cancer. Apparently a small adenoma requires 10 years or more to become cancerous, so taking aspirin on a regular basis may help during the earliest small-adenoma stage of colorectal cancer.

Researchers are trying to figure out an aspirin dosage that has positive effects for the heart and colon, but minimizes the tendency to cause stomach upset and bleeding. One recommendation for people with increased risk for colorectal cancer is to take a single 325-mg. aspirin tablet every other day (this amount is also in the range that has been suggested to reduce the incidence of cardiovascular disease).

For more information:

American Institute for Cancer Research
1-800-843-8114
www.aicr.org

National Cancer Institute/Cancer Information Service
(Answers questions from the public.)
1-800-422-6237
800-4-CANCER
www.cancernet.nci.nih.gov

National Cancer Institute/cancer trials information center
(Information on understanding trials, deciding whether to participate in trials, finding specific trials, plus research news and other resources.)
www.cancertrials.nci.nih.gov

American Cancer Society
1-800-227-2345
www.cancer.org

 **Chapter 2**

The Diet and Colon Cancer Connection

O ver the past few decades, researchers have been scrambling to make advances to treat cancer and understand what causes it. So far, we know many factors may cause cancer, but they are not completely understood. What makes the situation more complicated is that these factors are most likely interrelated. Can living "right" have an impact on our cancer risk?

A recent landmark report from the American Institute for Cancer Research (*Food Nutrition and the Prevention of Cancer— A Global Perspective*) estimates that:

- Eating the recommended five servings of fruits and vegetables each day can reduce cancer rates by more than 20 percent.
- Eating right, plus staying physically active and maintaining a healthy weight can cut cancer risk by 30 to 40 percent.
- Recommended dietary choices coupled with not smoking have the potential to reduce cancer risk by 60 to 70 percent.

Diet can play a role at any stage of cancer

What we eat (diet) is considered to be a factor in 20 to 50 percent of all cancer cases in general. Diet can play a role at any stage of cancer—initiation, promotion, or recovery. But here's the key—dietary components can have a protective role and help prevent cancer or they can have a stimulatory role and help promote cancer. It depends on the dietary component and the type of cancer.

Different food components appear to be more related to cancer prevention or promotion in certain organs. We'll look at colon cancer specifically in a bit, but for overall cancer prevention these are generally the foods to choose:

- Cruciferous (cabbage family) vegetables. These contain many phytochemicals with protective powers, such as bioflavonoids which are associated with a lower risk of colorectal cancer.
- Antioxidant-rich plant foods. This group includes foods rich in the carotenoid family of phytochemicals, vitamin C, vitamin E, and selenium, which help reduce damage to tissues from oxygen-seeking free radicals. It's the yellow, orange, and dark green vegetables that tend to be good sources of carotenoids. The citrus fruits, berries, and dark green vegetables are high in vitamin C. Whole grains are sources of vitamin E and selenium.
- High-fiber foods.

Overall these are the food habits to lose:

- High levels of food fat.
- High levels of alcohol.
- Extra (unneeded) calories.
- Nitrosamines (created when meats are fried or charcoal-broiled at very high temperatures; broiling, baking, stewing, and microwaving do not produce the same effect).

Beyond diet, age, genetics, and lifestyle (smoking, stress, lack of exercise, and environmental factors such as sun exposure and pollution) are also important things to consider.

What are free radicals and how are they made?

Free radicals are oxygen molecules and other highly reactive compounds that can damage body cells. It is believed that repeated assaults from various environmental factors (such as viruses, malnutrition, pollutants, or solar radiation) and normal cell production and division can cause free radicals to be produced in the body.

What can we do to defend ourselves against damage from free radicals?

Antioxidants from the food we eat help neutralize free radicals. There are an estimated 4,000 compounds in the foods we eat that act as antioxidants. The most known are vitamins C and E, beta carotene, and the mineral selenium. Researchers have been finding that a large group of colorful pigments in fruits and vegetables may be responsible for much of the antioxidant protection against free radicals. These antioxidants sacrifice themselves chemically to neutralize the free radicals so they can't cause oxidative damage to body cells (that's why they are called "anti" oxidants). Laboratory tests have concluded that blueberries, strawberries and concord grape juice have the highest antioxidant capacity.

Why is it important to protect ourselves against free radicals as we age?

Your body has a network of defenses set up to help neutralize free radicals so they can't cause trouble, but these defenses may become less efficient with age, allowing damage to accelerate.

To put the odds in your favor we are basically saying:

- Eat a diet rich in a variety of plant foods (fruits, vegetables, grains, and beans).
- Avoid eating a high fat diet.
- Exercise regularly.
- Achieve and maintain a healthy weight.
- Limit alcohol if you drink.
- Refrain from smoking.

What about colon cancer specifically?

There are common sense diet and lifestyle guidelines to help put the odds in your favor for all types of cancer. But each cancer seems to have its own subtle differences. Some cancers appear to be more related to diet or lifestyle than others, and some diet practices seem to have a stronger effect in some cancers than others.

Some researchers estimate that half of all colorectal cancers may be caused by inherited defects. The rest arise because of carcinogenic substances inhaled, swallowed, or bred by the bacteria that thrive in the colon.

Carcinogens in the colon

The food waste from our meals (what is left after the small intestine has absorbed all it can absorb) travels through the colon, then the rectum, then out of the body. This waste can contain different carcinogens. Plant foods in our diet help us counteract these carcinogens by decreasing the number, concentration, and exposure of these carcinogens to our colorectal cells.

The start of cancer in the colon

Colorectal tumors develop inside the colon or rectum. After the tumor has been there for a certain amount of time, some of its cells may break away and enter the bloodstream or lymph system. These cells may then form new tumors in other parts of the body.

There are some growths in the colon or rectum that are considered benign (not cancerous) tumors or polyps. But it is still important to remove these because they can bleed or interfere with the intestine's function, and may become cancerous over time if they are not removed.

Bile acids

When you eat fat in food, a greenish liquid called bile (bile contains cholesterol, lecithin, and bile acids and is made in the liver) is released into your small intestine to help with the digestion and absorption of fat. As much as you might not want your body to digest the fat you eat, it tries to digest as much as possible. Bile acids help transform the fat (triglycerides) into small droplets so they can be more available to the enzymes that are trying to break them down for absorption.

These bile acids may be left behind in the intestines. Unfriendly bacteria can convert bile acids into different carcinogenic forms. Whether or not these carcinogenic forms of bile acids actually do some damage depends on their concentration in the colon, and how quickly they move through the colon. The faster, the better, which is where your food choices can help. You can eat foods that encourage a lower concentration of the secondary bile acids, (avoiding high fat meals) and you can eat foods that speed up the colon (eating less fat and more plant foods and fiber).

The more fat you eat, the higher the concentration of bile acids collecting in your colon because bile acids are released expressly to help the body digest food fat. Too much fat and too little fiber in your diet means that food waste tends to travel slowly through your colon.

Eating lots of plant foods helps balance out the bile acids because they contain fiber, which speeds up the colon. Plant foods also contain antioxidants and helpful phytochemicals that help protect the colon cells from the carcinogens produced during digestion.

How big a difference can fiber make?

Let's put it this way, in a typical American diet (low in fiber) food takes three or more days to pass completely through the gastrointestinal tract and out of the body. With a higher fiber diet, food waste is eliminated in a day or two.

Let's review:

Fat is slow. Fiber is fast. High-fat, low-fiber diets tend to slow down the colon. Lower-fat, higher-fiber diets tend to speed it up.

How the food we eat helps the colon

Helpful nutrients from food, such as vitamins, minerals, and phytochemicals are absorbed into our bloodstream. High levels of these nutrients can help keep your body and immune system ready to fight potentially carcinogenic reactions.

But it's the materials that our body can't digest and absorb (food waste) that actually travel through and come in harmful contact with colon cells. The plant foods we eat (part of which is not absorbed) can then help to:

- Decrease the number of carcinogens.
- Decrease the concentration of carcinogens to colorectal cells.
- Decrease the exposure of these carcinogens to colorectal cells.

Colon 101

Just so we're all on the same page. To understand how the foods we eat can influence colon cancer risk, it helps to understand the basics of how the colon works:

Before the colon...

Once the stomach has broken down food, it releases small amounts of it into the small intestine. The bulk of the digesting and absorbing of the nutrients and calories from the food we eat happens in the small intestine. Carbohydrates are broken down into sugars and absorbed. Protein is broken down into amino acids and absorbed. Fat is broken down into fatty acids and glycerol, then absorbed. Vitamins and minerals, along with other important nutrients from the foods we eat, are absorbed. Fiber is one thing that does not get absorbed. The pancreas releases enzymes to help further digest food. Bile from the gallbladder and liver helps to break down fat in particular.

In the colon

The main job of the colon is to reabsorb water and salts as the food waste travels through it. This helps form solid stools, which can then exit the body after a couple of days, via the rectum (easily and without discomfort).

Nerves, hormones and electrical activity in the colon control these "movements." Muscles in the colon help propel the food waste slowly toward the rectum. "Normal" bowel movements range from three stools a day to as few as three a week.

The colon cells

Abnormal growths in the colon can become cancerous because:

- Like any genetically defective cells, the adenoma becomes more vulnerable to further mutation.
- With each meal or snack, colon cells are in direct contact with food waste. This contact accelerates carcinogenesis. Since we eat around the clock, colon cells are being hit and pushed continually.

Why the colon?

Why does cancer occur more often in the colon than other parts of the gastrointestinal tract?

- Food spends a much shorter time in the early portion of the gastrointestinal tract than in the colon. Any food carcinogens that are present are usually hidden until they reach the colon.
- The cells lining the colon divide at a rapid pace. With each division, errors (mutations) occur while copying DNA (the genetic blueprint). When the genes that regulate the timing of cell multiplication mutate, a colon cell may begin an out-of-control growth, which develops into a tumor or adenoma over time. This begins as a benign or harmless colon growth but is one step closer to becoming cancer because:

1. Genetically defective cells (like the adenoma) become more vulnerable to mutation.
2. Cells in the colon are continually bombarded by the concentration of waste from the digestive process, which accelerates carcinogenisis (the development of cancer).

• Carcinogens from food, free radicals, hormones, and other cancer promoters are all passing through the colon, potentially mutating genes of surrounding colon cells.

Questioning the fiber connection

For years there has been strong evidence that a high fiber, low fat diet reduces the risk of colon cancer. The *New England Journal of Medicine* reported in 1999 that several recent studies on fiber and colon cancer raise the question of whether the fiber element of the equation is related at all. Researchers at Harvard University and the Brigham and Women's Hospital in Boston looked at data from the Nurses' Health Study and found that nurses who ate 35 grams of fiber a day didn't have colon cancer any less than women who ate 13 grams a day (340: 169-76). Another study found similar results in men.

National Cancer Institute researcher Elaine Lanza suggests that the U.S. diet does not have the same range of fiber as the African diet (*The Lancet* Jan 30, 1999 vol. 353 p385 [1]), which suggested (years ago) a link between a high fiber diet and a very low incidence of colon cancer. Even the group of people who took in the highest amount of fiber in America did not meet the amount of fiber typically consumed on a daily basis in parts of Africa.

Researchers admit that the link between fiber and colon cancer is complex, and that they have yet to sort it out. However, people should still eat more high fiber foods, because they are an important source of other nutrients, and can lower the risk of heart attack, digestive problems, and possibly other forms of cancer.

The fat connection

There are at least 14 case-control studies that have explored the association of cancer risk with meat or fat consumption. A smaller number have looked at amounts of protein and calories. There are also several cohort studies going on right now.

Does the colon treat all fat equally?

So far some studies are saying no. There are studies that suggest that fats high in omega-3 fatty acids (found in fish, flaxseed, and various plant sources), monounsaturated fats, and omega-9 fatty acids (found in olive and canola oils and avocado) have no tumor-enhancing effects on the colon. Some European studies even suggest that monounsaturated fats may actually offer a protective effect against colon cancer.

The flip side is the omega-6 fatty acids (found in corn, safflower, and sunflower oils). Evidence suggests that too much omega-6 in the diet will increase the synthesis of prostaglandin E2, which can act as a cancer promoter. There are other fatty acids that tend to form prostaglandin E2 when you eat them in large amounts—and you'll find them in red meat. More on this in food steps 3 and 4 in Chapter 4.

- Membranes with omega-3 fatty acids are thought to be more resistant to cancer causing agents than membranes high in omega-6 fatty acids.
- Hormones produced from omega-3s have been tagged by researchers as more cancer protective than the same types of hormones made from omega-6s.

This is how I look at it. The typical American diet is so much higher in omega-6 than omega-3. I just concentrate on switching to omega-3 sources whenever possible. Most of the food products (and possibly restaurant foods) out there use one of the omega-6 vegetable oils, so I'm sure I get plenty of those already. What I can do at home is make sure I'm trying to balance them out by using low omega-6 oils for cooking (olive and canola). I make sure I eat a few servings of fish weekly and some flaxseed daily.

Is there a calcium connection?

Population studies have linked high rates of colon (and breast) cancer to low levels of calcium and vitamin D (we get both of these when we consume vitamin D fortified dairy products). When researchers tested vitamin D alone, it slowed cell growth. It is possible we will find out somewhere down the line that vitamin D has its own cancer-fighting properties. As a result, calcium may be important to colon cancer prevention for two reasons:

- One of its functions in the body is allowing the cells that line the colon to reproduce normally. If we don't have enough calcium, the cells lining the colon may multiply abnormally.
- When calcium meets up with bile acids left over from digestion and food-derived fats that didn't get absorbed and ended up in the colon (roughly about 5 percent of the food fats we eat aren't absorbed in the small intestine), they combine to make a harmless, soap-like substance.

Just remember that in order to help this beneficial "binding" process along, be sure to get the calcium you should be getting normally to help build and maintain bones, and to prevent osteoporosis.

What's the bottom line?

Experts still have questions about exactly how and why diet affects colorectal cancer development. Many scientists agree that diets low in fiber, high in fat and calories, and lacking in fruits and vegetables increase colon cancer risk. However, we do not yet know exactly how they influence cancer or the weighted importance of each of these dietary factors.

Whereas fat may promote colon cancer by increasing the concentration of bile acids in the intestine, fiber is thought to lower the concentration of bile acids along with other carcinogens that might be in the intestine. Fruits and vegetables contribute fiber, vitamins, minerals, and other compounds (such as phytochemicals) that may help counteract the effects of carcinogens.

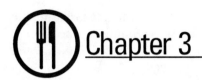 Chapter 3

Everything You Ever Wanted to Ask Your Dietitian About Preventing Colon Cancer

Q **What if my diet is high in fiber, fruits, and vegetables, and lower in fat, saturated fat, red or processed meat, sugar, and alcohol? How much would it help reduce my risk?**

We don't quite know what the diet-related portion of risk is. Scientists do estimate that up to 75 percent of all cases of colorectal cancer could be prevented through following a mostly plant-based diet, maintaining a healthy body weight, keeping physically active, and not smoking (American Institute for Cancer Research, Diet, Nutrition, and Cancers of the Colon and Rectum, updated 2000).

Q **What is fiber, exactly?**

Often called "roughage," fiber is any part of a plant food that does not break down during digestion. There are two types of fiber: insoluble and soluble.

Water-soluble fiber dissolves in water to make a gel-like material. It is found in oats, barley, psyllium, beans, some fruits, vegetables and nuts). Water-soluble fiber delays digestion and slows the movement of partly digested food through the small intestine.

Insoluble fiber is not able to dissolve in water. It speeds up the movement of partly digested food and is found in wheat bran, whole grain breads, vegetables, and fruits with edible skins and seeds, such as strawberries and tomatoes.

Q **Is it still possible that a high-fiber diet may help reduce the risk of colon cancer?**
Despite the two studies in April and May 2000 from the *New England Journal of Medicine* that blasted the benefits of fiber, I think it is. Some researchers say the studies do suggest that fiber won't protect against colon cancer.

Between two groups of men and women, 35 years and older, studies found that there wasn't a difference in the amount of new polyps found four years after the individuals had pre-cancerous polyps removed from their colons. One group ate a low-fat diet with 5 to 8 servings of fruits and vegetables a day, (averaging 35 grams of fiber a day) and the other group ate more red meat, fewer beans, and less fish (averaging 20 grams of fiber a day).

These results tell us that fiber doesn't seem to inhibit the formation of polyps. So if fiber doesn't inhibit polyps, can it still help prevent colon cancer? Quite possibly, and here's why:

Earlier we learned that only a certain percentage of formed polyps go on to become cancerous, which traditionally takes 10 years or so. This was a four-year study. The study did not measure whether there was a smaller percentage of cancerous polyps after 10 or more years. It did not measure mortality from colon cancer over 10 to 20 years. Case in point: When you stop smoking, it can take 10 years to see a difference in your risk of lung cancer. One colon cancer researcher, John Potter of the University of Washington, stated that the process of developing polyps or cancer may take many years, even though polyps themselves become visible over a relatively short period of time.

So don't throw away your raisin bran just yet. Researchers remind us that fiber definitely benefits us in other ways. Solid research links a high-fiber diet to lower blood pressure, decreased blood cholesterol levels, and reduced risk of developing type 2 diabetes.

Q How much fiber should my kids and I get every day?
The National Cancer Institute recommends 20 to 30 grams of fiber a day for adults. I would definitely shoot for 30 grams a day. Generally young people, ages three to 18 years should take in daily fiber equal to, or greater than their age, plus 5 grams. A 10-year-old would shoot for a total of 15 grams, for example. Of course, it's always a good idea to check with a health professional if you have special dietary needs or medical conditions.

Q Does the way we cook or grill food have anything to do with colon cancer risk?
A diet high in grilled or barbecued meat may increase the risk of colorectal and stomach cancers. This is because cooking meat, poultry, or fish at high temperatures, especially over an open flame, can cause cancer-promoting substances to form on the meat. I personally like my meat on the burned side, which is not a good thing when done often.

In general, high temperature cooking produces substances that may cause cancer. Cooking in hot fat generally occurs at a higher temperature than other methods. So cooking at lower temperatures (baking, boiling, braising, microwaving, poaching, roasting, steaming, stewing, and using a slow cooker) will definitely help.

When you do grill

What can you do when you want to grill? Grab a marinade and run with it. Research shows that marinating foods, regardless of the marinade ingredients or length of marinating time, greatly reduces the production of carcinogenic compounds in meats cooked at high temperatures. Here are some tips for safe grilling:

- Use marinades, preferably those with canola oil, olive oil, or no fat.
- Trim off fat before you grill the meat. (Choose lean meats whenever possible.)
- Pre-cook meats in the oven or microwave, then grill briefly just for added flavor.
- Flip meats with a spatula or use tongs instead of a fork. (Juices are less likely to ooze out and drip onto the coals, causing flare-ups.)

- Do not squirt starter fluid into coals while meats are cooking. (Keep a water spray bottle handy.)
- Avoid placing meat directly over coals.
- Resist eating charred meat or remove charred parts before eating.

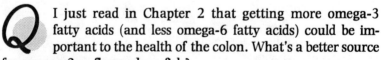 **Are nitrosamines something I should be worried about?** Nitrosamines are known to have carcinogenic activity. They are formed during the breakdown of nitrites and nitrates, which are the chemicals actually added by manufacturers to cure and preserve the meat. They give cured meats a pink look, and protect against potentially deadly botulism. In the 1970s, scientists detected nitrosamines in many popular foods (cooked bacon and sausage, cured pork and dried beef, etc.) Bacon had one of the highest levels of nitrosamines of them all.

But here's the great news. If you happen to love bacon and hot dogs, there are a few different substances that actually help stop the formation of nitrosamines (from the nitrates and nitrites). For example, some meat-product companies have already been adding them to their products:

- Vitamins C and E (antioxidants). (You won't see this on the label, you will likely see their chemical names, "ascorbic acid," "ascorbate," or "tocopherol.")
- P-coumaric and chlorogenic acids (found in fruits and vegetables).

If your favorite turkey, bacon, and hot dogs don't have one of the above in its list of ingredients, you can always eat them with a good dose of citrus fruits or green vegetables.

I just read in Chapter 2 that getting more omega-3 fatty acids (and less omega-6 fatty acids) could be important to the health of the colon. What's a better source for omega-3s—flaxseed or fish? In addition to omega-3s, fish gives you protein and the antioxidant selenium. Ground flaxseed gives you soluble fiber and some phytoestrogens. Eating fish a couple of times a week sounds reasonable to me (then again, I'm a fish lover). Adding a couple of teaspoons of ground flaxseed to my oatmeal or smoothie a few times a week is just something extra I like to do. To me, they go together. I also use olive oil (which doesn't contain omega-6 fatty acids) and canola oil (which contains some omega-3s and less omega-6s than similar neutral tasting oils) in cooking, instead of the omega-6 rich vegetable oils (corn, safflower, and sunflower).

Q **I'm eating healthy and exercising, so why am I not losing weight?**

If you are exercising regularly and strength training as well, you are probably adding muscle weight while   decreasing some body fat. Remember, muscle weighs more than body fat. Your weight could very well stay the same even though you are building muscle and losing body fat. Keep in mind that you are healthier for it.

You could also consider portion sizes. It is possible, even if you are choosing healthful foods, that the portions may be too large for your caloric needs. If you keep this up, your won't see any actual lost pounds. Or, if you eat out often, you may be eating more calories and grams of fat than you realize.

Q **Do the high-protein, low-carbohydrate fad diets help you lose weight? Are there any risks?**

Anytime a high-protein, low carbohydrate-eating plan is recommended, it is not intended for long-term use. Carbohydrates are the preferred fuel source for the body. When the body uses protein for energy, nitrogen must be removed first. Extra nitrogen must be removed from the body (via urine) because too much circulating in the blood is toxic. This can overtax the kidneys. Anyone with impaired kidney function should avoid a high-protein diet.

Here's one weight loss fact you should always remember. Fat gets stored in the body when the calories we take in are higher than the calories we are burning, regardless of where those calories come from—even from protein or carbs.

The long-term effects of high-protein fad diets have not been studied. Many people will lose weight on these plans because they are mostly low-calorie plans. By limiting carbohydrates, they are forcing the followers to limit portion size. The weight loss has more to do with the decrease in total calories and forced portion sizing rather the fact that the diet is high in protein. How healthy and permanent the weight loss is on this plan remains to be proven. I have met several people who lost weight on one of these high-protein plans. None of them maintained the lost weight—each is back to where he started.

Q **Are high-protein diets more healthful than high-carbohydrate diets?**

No! But hopefully, the high-carbohydrate diet is nicely balanced with some protein, fat, and mostly complex carbohydrates (whole grains, vegetables, beans, and fruits) with little sugar. Don't forget that there are many important nutrients (such as fiber) in carbohydrate-rich foods (grains, fruits, vegetables, and beans) that are absent in the high-protein plans. High-protein diets are often high in saturated fat too. Most people can't even follow them for more than a few months because they are too difficult to keep up. There is no evidence that individuals who lose weight on such diets maintain their weight loss.

Q **I keep hearing about carbohydrates...the addict's diet, refined, complex, simple...what do I need to know?**

Don't be swayed by any anti-carbohydrate rhetoric. What gets lost in this message is that there are different types of carbohydrates, and you can't just toss sugar into the same nutritional camp as broccoli or whole wheat bread. Certainly, no one has evidence that we shouldn't be eating whole grains, beans, or fruits and vegetables. Now, lots of soda, fat-free high sugar cookies, and processed grains...that's another story. Here are some definitions to help you sift through the information.

Simple carbohydrates: Single sugar molecules or parts of sugar molecules bonded together. These single sugars are the building blocks for all carbohydrates. Naturally occurring sugars are glucose, fructose, or galactose. Table sugar is sucrose and lactose bonded together. Lactose, the sugar found in milk, is also made of two sugars (glucose and galactose). Simple carbohydrates are digested rapidly to form glucose molecules.

Complex carbohydrates: Long strands of sugar molecules linked together. They take longer to break down to glucose. Bread, pastas, grain-based foods, and starchy vegetables like potatoes and corn are excellent sources of complex carbohydrates.

Refined carbohydrates: Have had certain components of the plant removed, usually the germ and bran. Both simple and complex carbohydrates can be refined. Table sugar is refined from raw sugar. White flour is refined from whole wheat grain. Even fruit juice is refined if pulp and fiber have been removed.

It makes sense to emphasize the complex, unrefined carbohydrates. They contain the germ of the grain, which contains essential vitamins and helpful oils. They also contain the bran, which contributes fiber and phytochemicals. Generally, the higher the fiber in a carbohydrate, the more complex the carbohydrate is, and the slower it converts from carbohydrate eaten to glucose in the blood. This helps most people maintain consistent blood sugar levels at the very least.

Q I've heard about cancer prevention benefits of garlic. Should I be taking garlic supplements?

Scientists are still hammering out the health benefits of garlic and other vegetables in the onion family. Certainly, enjoying the onion family in homemade meals and "food to go" is a great idea and fairly easy to do if you like them, but supplements? I wouldn't take them. You need to know that all the various and sundry forms of garlic supplements on the market are not regulated. What they are made of, and how much actual allyl sulfides (the phytochemical thought to be one of the helpful plant agents) can vary. Also, keep in mind that each batch of garlic differs in its chemical content due to growing conditions and individual strains of garlic. If you don't like the taste of garlic, try roasting a few bulbs of it. Cut off the tops of the garlic bulb, set in on a sheet of foil, drizzle the top with a little olive oil, then wrap in foil. Roast in an oven at 300 degrees for about 40 minutes. The flavor really mellows when you cook it this way.

There are other members in the garlic family that you might like (for example, shallots and onions).

 I know I should be eating more fruits and vegetables, but should I be worried about pesticide residues and cancer risk?

Some experts say that less than 1 percent of all cancers are attributed to pesticides and other manufactured chemicals in air, water, soil, and food. Compare this figure with the estimated 60 to 70 percent of all cancers linked to lifestyle factors you can control and it doesn't seem like much of a concern.

Don't get me wrong; it is still a must to wash all produce thoroughly in water, scrubbing the skin, removing outer leaves when possible. This not only reduces pesticide residues but also gets rid of dirt and bacteria that could make you sick. I generally try to buy seasonal produce and not rely too heavily on imported grapes and other fruits coming from countries with more lax food safety and pesticide regulations. That just makes good sense to me.

I was surprised to read in a report from Consumers' Union (*Consumer Reports*, March 1999) that according to their findings, more pesticide residues were found on domestic produce than on imports, except for imported grapes, tomatoes, and carrots (something to keep in mind). Recently a panel of experts from the U.S. and Canada reviewed more than 50 studies and concluded the benefits of eating fruits and vegetables far outweigh the potential risks from pesticides.

That doesn't mean we shouldn't try to avoid pesticides. The effect of pesticides on the human body is not entirely known. Perhaps more importantly, we know little about how they might interact with each other. This could be a reason that you see more and more organic produce available. You may wonder which fruits and vegetables would we reap the biggest benefits from buying organic, and which are more pesticide prone. Two reports came out in 1999, one from the Environmental Working Group, a nonprofit consumer organization, and one from Consumers'

Union. Their rankings of fruits and vegetables with the highest pesticide residues didn't exactly parallel, but between the two of them, there is a loose list of produce that you might want to consider buying organic, if available and affordable. The Consumers' Union (*Consumer Reports*, March 1999) and the Environmental Working Group (February 1999) both found apples, spinach, peaches, pears, grapes, celery, and green beans as having the highest pesticide residues.

The Consumers' Union listed tomatoes, lettuce, and carrots as having a "dishonorable mention," whereas the Environmental Working Group didn't list any of them in their "terrible 10." The Environmental Working Group listed strawberries and potatoes in their "terrible 10," although Consumers' Union didn't list them.

 What can I do at home to reduce my pesticide intake from produce?

- Buy organic versions of the more pesticide-prone produce listed above when available and affordable.
- Thoroughly wash fruits and vegetables with cool, running water, scrubbing when needed.
- Throw away the outer leaves of lettuce and greens, where pesticide residues tend to be higher.
- Peel the pesticide-prone produce items, especially when serving them to children.

Which cancers have the strongest associations with what you eat?

Reducing risk through diet changes is thought to have the strongest associations with breast, colon/rectum, and prostate cancers (*Cancer*, 1998; 83:1425-32).

Many of the food suggestions to help prevent colon cancer involve eating more plant foods and less animal foods, particularly red meat. Does this type of diet give me enough protein?

In America, protein tends to be overrated. Most Americans get more than two times the protein they actually need. Too much protein may even be linked to a variety of health problems. Scientists used to think you needed to eat plant proteins, which complemented each other to make "complete" proteins, in the same meal. We now know this complementing takes place over many hours. By eating a variety of plant-based foods every day, you will get the building blocks (essential amino acids) you need for growth and good health.

Q Do you have another question?
Do you have a question on diet and colon cancer that isn't answered in this or the following chapter? There are a few great places to go with your questions. You'll find a list of helpful organizations at the end of Chapter 1 (page 18).

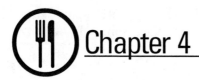 Chapter 4

10 Food Steps to Freedom

P eople say, "It's all in the genes, so there's nothing I can do anyway." In one sense, it's true for many diseases; there is a portion of risk going directly back to the family tree. But there is another portion of risk that has to do with the way we live and eat. We can't do anything about our genes but we can do something about these other possible risks.

For years now cancer experts have reported that the three cancers most likely to be linked to our diet are cancers of the prostate, colon, and breast (book three in the "Tell Me What to Eat" series covers what we know about helping prevent breast cancer). The scientific evidence on how what we eat can influence our risk of developing certain cancers keeps growing every year.

You've read about the scientific connection between diet and colon cancer in Chapter 2. Now we are going to put it together, along with recent research clues, and come up with 10 food steps to freedom. These are 10 food steps you can take today to reduce your risk of colon cancer in the future.

No miracle foods for cancer

There are no miracle foods for cancer prevention. But there is a connection between diet and cancer prevention. That's all we have right now—evidence giving us links and associations between the two. Some of this scientific evidence does come from animal studies, which may or may not apply to humans. With every study, we get closer and closer to putting this puzzle together. Right now, as I see it, we have some of the puzzle assembled and we are starting to see a picture.

So what I'm saying is, this is not about miracle foods, it's about common-sense steps you can take today to put the odds in your favor. It's like taking out some insurance. You may not need it, and it may not be exactly the right policy, but it isn't going to hurt, and it will most likely help you in the long run. After all, we are talking about simple steps, like eating more fruits, vegetables, whole grains, and fish, and eating less red meat, total fat, saturated fat, sugar, and alcohol. It's not a sure thing by any means. Nothing is when it comes to preventing cancer. But it's a chance most of us will choose to take, especially because following these 10 food steps to freedom will also help reduce your risk of heart disease, high blood pressure, diabetes, and other cancers.

Step 1: Eat 5 to 10 servings of fruits and vegetables a day

The benefit of fiber to colon cancer risk reduction is up for debate for the moment (see Chapter 3 for more on this). But the evidence on vegetables and colon cancer still stands strong. Vegetable consumption has shown the strongest and most consistent association with colon cancer risk reduction. One researcher reviewed 30 related studies in 1993 and found that more than 80 percent of the studies showed vegetables had a protective effect (*Epidemiological Review* 15:499, 1993).

What about fruit? Fruit has not been evaluated as thoroughly as vegetables alone or in combination with vegetables. Recent data suggest although fruits are protective, they aren't as protective as vegetables (*Gastroenterology Clinics of North America* 27:325, 1998).

You must resist the urge to take the vitamins found in vegetables in pill form (such as beta-carotene). It's the food itself that works, not necessarily one or two of the nutrients in the food. Fruits and vegetables also contain an array of other nutrients and phytochemicals that most likely work best together.

(Phytochemicals are compounds found in plants that do not have an established nutrient effect, but nonetheless could decrease the risk of cancer through a variety of mechanisms.)

Researchers have been finding that a large group of colorful pigments in fruits and vegetables may be responsible for much of the antioxidant protection against free radicals. Laboratory tests have been done to find out what the total antioxidant capacities of specific fruits and vegetables are. Of the ones tested thus far, blueberries, strawberries, and concord grape juice scored highest.

Phytochemicals with anticancer properties

Which phytochemicals have anticancer effects? A few that we already know for sure are allyl sulfides in the garlic/onion family, and the isothiocynates and indoles in broccoli and other cabbage family vegetables. For example, although still considered preliminary, studies have shown a link between high consumption of garlic and reduced rates of colorectal cancer (along with breast and stomach cancer). A study on lutein-rich fruits and vegetables (spinach, broccoli, lettuce, greens, brussels sprouts, and peas) showed that people who reported eating the most foods rich in lutein were much less likely to develop colon cancer than those eating fewer lutein-rich foods. For other potentially helpful phytochemicals, see the table on pages 42 and 43.

Let's not forget the antioxidants

Foods rich in antioxidants have been linked to a lower risk of colon cancer. Notice it says "foods" rich in antioxidants and not "pills." Results from a four-year study showed that taking antioxidant supplements (containing beta-carotene and vitamins E and C) did not reduce a person's risk of developing colorectal cancer, but that people who ate foods high in antioxidants had a lower tendency of developing them (*Tufts University Diet & Nutrition Letter*, Sept. 1994 vol. 12 n7 p1[1]).

Ten to 20 years ago studies suggested that three antioxidants might relate to colon cancer risk:

- High levels of foods with vitamin C decreased the number of recurrent polyps in the colon.

Helpful Phytochemicals

Phytochemical	Food source	How it might work
*Allyl sulfides (allium family)	garlic, onions, scallions, chives, leeks, shallots	Lab tests have found they may: 1) increase production of enzymes that help rid the body of carcinogens, 2) depress the growth of human cancer cells, 3) block the production of the potentially carcinogenic nitrosamines (garlic).
*Antioxidants	fruits, vegetables legumes	Silence free radicals that directly attack DNA.
Beta Carotene	apricots, cantaloupe, mangoes, carrots, pumpkin, winter squash sweet potatoes, dark green vegetables, greens and all fruits	May reduce the risk of some cancers by protecting cells from damage.
*Caffeic acidin	all fruit	Makes carcinogens soluble (dissolvable in water) and easily removed from cells.
Capsaicin	chili peppers	
*Ellagic acid	fruits (red grapes, berries)	Protects DNA from mutation.
*Ferulic acid	all fruits	Prevents conversion of nitrates to carcinogenic nitrosamines.
Flavonoids		Give antioxidant protection against free radicals or may curtail cell growth and keep toxic substances from reaching cells.
*Folic acid	legumes, fruits and vegetables	Corrects DNA errors and controls the number of mutations.
Genistein	soybeans	

Helpful Phytochemicals (cont.)

Phytochemical	Food source	How it might work
Indoles	cruciferous/cabbage family vegetables	May inhibit growth of estrogen sensitive human breast cells
Isoflavones	beans	Acts as an antioxiant.
*Isothiocyanates	cruciferous/cabbage family vegetables	Trigger enzymes that block carcinogens.
*Lutein (a carotenoid)	spinach, broccoli lettuce, tomatoes, oranges, carrots, celery, greens	Not sure, but lutein, like other carotenoids, is an antioxidant that may destroy free radicals.
Limonene	citrus fruits, other fruits and vegetables	Appears to have a blocking effect against carcinogenesis.
Phytates	whole grains	Bind free iron molecules remaining in the colon following a meal. (Free iron has the potential to make free radicals.)
*Phytosterols	legumes fruits and vegetables whole grains	Block the harmful effects of secondary bile acids on the colon cells.
Protease Inhibitors	beans	Inhibits induced tumors in many organ sites
Resveratrol	purple-red grapes	Extremely potent against cancer cells in laboratory tests.
*Sulforaphane	broccoli and other cabbage family vegetable	Appears to trigger production of enzymes in the body's cells that help rid the body of cancer-causing agents.

* Phytochemicals that seem to help protect against colon cancer.

- Animals eating large amounts of vitamin E had fewer tumors.
- Selenium intake in 27 countries was related to colon cancer. The more selenium consumed, the lower the colon cancer rates were.

Another potential benefit to fruits and vegetables: fiber and folate!

I know you've been hearing about fiber off and on through the book so far. However, epidemiological studies have shown repeatedly that a low total fat, high fiber diet is associated with a lower incidence of colon cancer. A Harvard Medical School study in 1992 found that men whose daily fiber intake was about 30 grams had a reduced likelihood of developing pre-cancerous colon changes as they aged. Eating at least five servings of fruits and vegetables a day is a quick way to get 15 grams of fiber (half of the 30 gram goal).

In terms of the antioxidant-like vitamin, folate (folic acid), some evidence is suggesting it may be linked to the prevention of colorectal cancer. Folate can be found in certain vegetables and fruits (as well as whole grains and beans).

Tips to take home:

- Eat vegetables raw (if appropriate). Serve a nice plate of raw vegetables with a favorite reduced calorie bottled salad dressing, or make a quick dip with a favorite light or fat-free sour cream blended with Hidden Valley Ranch dip powder.
- When you cook vegetables, microwave them in 1/4 cup of water or steam them only until they are al dente (just tender but still firm to the bite). You will be more likely to eat and enjoy vegetables if they aren't overcooked or canned (some of which can have an off flavor and texture).
- For convenience, always have bags of your favorite vegetables in your freezer. This way on those nights when you are pulling dinner together quickly you can just open up a bag of vegetables and micro-cook them quickly.
- Avoid peeling fruits and vegetables when you can (this saves time too), because eating the skin ensures that you get most of the fiber that they contain. Be sure to rinse them with warm water to remove surface dirt and any potential bacteria before eating.

- Whole fruits and vegetables contain more fiber than juice does. Not that juice is "bad." But you can't drink your way to five to 10 servings of fruits and vegetables a day. One or so of your servings can come from daily orange juice or carrot juice. I think this is a great and easy habit to get into. Pick juice with pulp when possible. The pulp is the part of the fruit that contains this fiber we are talking about.
- It's good to drink at least eight cups of water (and other fluids without caffeine) a day.
- Toss a handful of fruit on pancakes, waffles, french toast, yogurt, ice cream, and cereal.
- Add vegetables every chance you get—even on your pizza!
- Get dipping. Dip your vegetables in salad dressing (made with canola oil or olive oil) or ranch dip (made by blending your favorite light or nonfat sour cream with Hidden Valley Ranch dip powder).

Step 2: Eat cabbage family (cruciferous) vegetables several times a week

I know you just got through hearing about the importance of fruits and vegetables. But this food step is about one specific group of very powerful vegetables—the cabbage family vegetables. Study after study suggests that eating cabbage family (cruciferous) vegetables can lower the risk of developing colon cancer.

Cruciferous vegetables contribute known antioxidants such as vitamin C (which defend the body against compounds that can promote the growth of cancerous tumors), fiber, and powerful phytochemicals like indoles and sulforaphane. All of these things make cruciferous vegetables helpful.

What about phytochemicals?

Sulforaphane (found in large amounts in broccoli) appears to trigger production of special enzymes in the body's cells that help rid the body of cancer-causing agents. Johns Hopkins scientist Paul Talalay, M.D. suggests that sulforaphane blocks tumor formation in animals and presumably in humans.

The cabbage (cruciferous) family vegetables

Obviously the cabbage family includes cabbage and the nutritionally infamous broccoli, but what are the less common vegetables in this potentially protective family?

- Brussels sprouts.
- Cauliflower.
- Cabbage.
- Broccoli.
- Mustard greens.
- Kale.
- Kohlrabi.

(For shopping tips on the above cabbage family vegetables, see Chapter 7.)

Tips to take home:

- Raw broccoli and cauliflower florets might appeal to people who don't care for them cooked. Serve raw florets with vinaigrette (made with canola or olive oil) or ranch dip (reduced fat if desired).
- Raw shredded cabbage works great as an alternative to lettuce for some summer salad recipes (such as Chinese chicken salad or ramen noodle salad) and other recipes such as fish tacos.
- Add bite-sized broccoli and cauliflower florets to green salads whenever possible to boost the nutrients and get in a serving of cabbage family vegetables fairly unnoticeably.
- Have frozen assorted vegetable bags featuring broccoli and/or cauliflower on hand in your freezer. On busy nights, just pop some in the microwave.
- If you are having pasta, microwave some broccoli or cauliflower just until tender, then add them into your pasta and sauce. You'll barely notice them. This is an easy way to work in your cabbage family veggies. This even works great with macaroni and cheese!

- Add kale, kohlrabi, or cabbage to your favorite stir-fry recipes, perhaps instead of bok choy.
- Add any of the cabbage family vegetables to soups and stews when appropriate.
- Add any of the cabbage family vegetables to your favorite casserole recipes when appropriate.
- I haven't had much luck with frozen brussels sprouts tasting great, so you might want to make a point of enjoying them when they are in season.
- To cut corners, buy pre-washed, pre-shredded bags of cabbage for all your coleslaw, stir-fry, and dinner salad needs.

Step 3: Eat omega-3 rich fish several times a week

Omega-3 fatty acids have been shown to decrease the risk of heart attacks and are linked to lowering blood pressure and serum triglyceride levels, and helping prevent blood clots (thereby decreasing the chance of stroke). But research continues to show us that they can do much more.

Omega-3 fatty acids have been shown to slow or prevent the growth of certain cancers (in animal studies). They also reduce symptoms of inflammatory diseases (rheumatoid arthritis is shown to be less common in people with diets rich in omega-3 fatty acids). It is currently being investigated whether too little omega-3s may contribute to depression (omega-3s are important components of nerve cells) and impaired bone growth.

This sounds great if you happen to love fish. But what if you don't? Nature has provided a handful of plant foods that contain ALA (alpha-linolenic acid). The human body can convert some of this ALA into one of the omega-3 fatty acids found in fish (EPA, eicosapentaenoic acid).

How many servings of high omega-3 foods do we need to get some of the disease prevention benefits? Most experts recommend two to three servings of fish high in omega-3s per week as part of

15 Fabulous Fish Sources of Omega-3 fatty acids

	Serving size	Omega-3 (mg)	Calories
Sardines, canned in tomato sauce	2 sardines	1,424	135
Coho salmon[1] (steamed)	3 oz.	1,337	156
Pacific oysters	3 oz.	1,224	139
Sockeye salmon[1]	3 oz.	1,158	184
Mackerel, baked	3 oz.	1,118	223
Tuna steaks (blue fin) baked	3 oz.	1,106	156
Rainbow trout, wild, baked	3 oz.	999	128
Shark steaks, cooked	3 oz.	975	153
Albacore tuna (white tuna) (canned in water)	1/2 can	803	110
Pickled herring	2 oz.	788	148
Pink salmon, canned	3 oz.	755	118
Sea bass, baked	3 oz.	648	105
Shrimp, cooked	6 oz.	554	168
Halibut, baked	3 oz.	466	119
Anchovies, canned in oil (drained)	5 anchovies	414	42

Top 6 Plant Sources of Omega-3 fatty acids

	Serving size	ALA (mg)	Omega-3 (mg)	Calories
Flaxseed[2]	1 tbs.	2,175	0	59
Canola oil[3]	1 tbs.	1,302	0	123
Broccoli, raw	1 cup	114	0	25
Cantaloupe cubes	1 cup	107	0	56
Red kidney beans (canned)	1/2 cup	75	0	109
Spinach, raw	2 cups	70	0	13

[1]Farm-raised salmon has a little less omega-3 fatty acids than wild salmon, but is still considered a good source.

a varied diet. And eating more fish means we are more likely to be eating less red meat—which is food step 4.

Tips to take home:

- Switch to canola oil for cooking and baking when you can.
- Choose salad dressings, margarine, chips, and other food products that use canola oil and limit those products that contain the high omega-6 oils (corn, safflower, and sunflower oil).
- Consider adding the plant sources of omega-3s (broccoli, spinach, kidney beans, and flaxseed (if not allergic) to recipes whenever possible.
- Enjoy cantaloupe when it is in season. Make it a little fancy by tossing cantaloupe pieces with fresh or frozen blueberries or raspberries. Make a melon salad by mixing in some watermelon and/or honeydew melon.
- Enjoy a spinach salad with kidney beans, and broccoli florets dressed with a canola salad dressing. This adds four of these omega-3 plant foods to your day (see the recipe for omega-3 spinach salad in Chapter 6).
- Add a teaspoon of ground flaxseed to a smoothie, glass of juice, or bowl of cold or hot cereal a few times a week.

---

[2]To make the nutrients in flaxseed available to your body, it is important to grind them up first (in a coffee grinder, for example), then add them to your food or recipe. Store unused ground flaxseed in the refrigerator.

[3]Canola oil does contain twice the amount of omega-6 fatty acids than it does omega-3s but it still has the best ratio of omega-3 to omega-6 of any of the vegetable cooking oils.

Note: There are two plant foods known to have ALA that you won't find in this table (soybeans an walnuts) because they also contain significant amounts of omega-6 fatty acids. When eaten in much larger amounts than omega-3s, omega- 6s can decrease their beneficial effects. The highest omega-6 oils are corn and safflower. USDA food composition data was used to for this table.

- Use 1/4 to 1/2 cup of ground flaxseed instead of 1/4 to 1/2 cup of the flour called for when making a batch of homemade muffins or a loaf of bread. That way you will have about 1 1/2 to 3 teaspoons of flaxseed per serving or slice.

Step 4: Eat less red meat (and more beans!)

Some experts believe you can cut your colorectal risk in half just by reducing the amount of red meat you eat to one serving a day. How does this help protect the body? Experts aren't sure yet but some think it has something to do with undigested fat in the colon producing extra cancer-causing compounds. We also know that red meat is often high in saturated fat, which promotes tumors in the large intestine. If meat is cooked over high heat until charred, harmful chemicals form, and they are deposited back into the meat on the barbecue via rising smoke. (Furthermore, if we eat a lot of red meat, we are also not likely to be eating protective plant foods.)

Red meat does not contain the more desirable omega-3 and omega-9 fatty acids. In fact, red meat contains arachidonic acid. Too much of this fatty acid is thought to form prostalandin E2, which can act as a cancer promoter.

Excess iron is another possible connection. Red meat includes high amounts of iron. You were probably told to eat lots of it if you were anemic during a pregnancy. Recent studies have found a link between high levels of iron (in blood and in the food subjects ate) and colon cancer. Too much iron is never a good idea because it's a mineral. Our bodies can't get rid of any extra we could be taking in. Experts suspect that too much iron may increase the formation of free radicals. More free radicals mean more chance of damage to the body's DNA, which can lead to the development of some cancers.

Red meat is also high in protein. Some researchers have found links between high-protein diets and increased cancer risk. Right now, research is going on to find out how protein, fat, or a combination of the two might be linked to cancer risk.

Trading beef for beans

The typical American diet is focused on meat. But in some countries, like India and Mexico, beans appear daily in the traditional dishes people like to eat. My daughters love to eat Mexican beans and rice with dinner and they love chili too. I don't think Americans avoid beans on purpose, we just haven't gotten into the bean habit.

Believe me—the health benefits are there. Beans (legumes) are high in protein, folate, and dietary fiber. They are low in fat, and full of helpful phytochemicals. Kidney beans are one of the top plant sources of one of the omega-3 fatty acids.

When you do eat red meat...

Depending on where in this country you live, red meat could be the mainstay of almost every meal. Eating it less often is going to take some major motivation. That's what the following "tips to take home" will help you with. But what can we do when we do eat red meat to keep it as healthful as possible?

1. Cook it the lean way

- Trim off any visible fat from the meat before cooking. If it is a fattier cut of meat, you can then cook it on a rack so the fat drips away from the meat.
- Choose less fatty (or marbled) cuts of meat like the round, shank, tenderloin or sirloin in beef, or the center or tenderloin of pork.
- Cook your meat with a minimum of added fat. Try to avoid saturated fat, such as: shortening, butter, or the omega-6 vegetable oils (corn, safflower, and sunflower). If you do need to use some fat, switch to olive or canola oil if possible.
- When using a leaner cut, cooking it over low heat for a long period of time can be a great way to tenderize it. Cooking in a slow cooker works wonders. Roasting can also work well.

2. Eat smaller portions

- A healthful serving of meat is about the size of a deck of cards or about three ounces of boneless, cooked meat (four ounces before cooking). This is the size of a quarter pound hamburger patty. Some people may laugh at this amount, thinking: "I'm just getting started." That's why this could very well be the toughest food step for some people out there who have gotten into the blissful habit of eating huge meat servings.
- Eat more of the other meal components (fruits, vegetables, whole grains) to fill up on instead of the meat.
- Certain cuisine and recipes (pasta with meat sauce, beef and vegetable stir fry over rice, beef or pork chili with beans served with corn bread) normally use smaller amounts of meat. Meat is one of many ingredients in the dish instead of the main event. Try to enjoy these dishes more often.

Tips to take home:

- Don't go sitting down once a day to a 12-ounce steak. A serving of red meat is considered to be three ounces of cooked meat (the size of a deck of cards).
- Gravitate toward meat recipes that use meat as a garnish or one ingredient of many—rather than meat as the main event. Certain Japanese, Chinese, Vietnamese, Indian, African, and Mexican dishes are more likely to do this.
- Poultry and fish are good substitutes for red meat. Start trying and collecting fish and poultry recipes that are moderate in fat and call for canola or olive oil.
- Canned beans taste great, and they make cooking with beans a lot easier. Add canned beans to soups, stews, and all kinds of salads.
- A couple of times a week, substitute bean-based dishes (like bean burritos, rice and beans, mostly-bean chili, lentil soup) for dishes with lots of meat.
- Don't cook dried beans in the same water you soaked them in (to minimize gaseous side effects). And if

eating beans is uncomfortable for you, try the enzyme products available, like Beano or Say Yes To Beans, which help digest the fiber in beans so it doesn't cause problems for you.
- Drink at least eight cups of water a day.

Red meat tips
- Remove all visible fat before cooking meat (less to drip down onto the coals).
- Place a lid on the grill to moderate the cooking temperature.
- Partially precook the meat (microwave, bake, or broil), then finish cooking on the grill (this will reduce the meat's exposure to the heat).
- Avoid using mesquite, as soft wood produces extremely high heat.
- If the dripping fat creates smoke, reduce the heat. And do not eat the charred part of the meat.
- Nitrates used to cure meats can convert into carcinogenic nitrosamines in the stomach. Adding vitamin C to cured meat controls the production of these carcinogens.

Step 5: Eat less saturated fat and avoid eating a high-fat diet

Personally, I don't believe that eating a very low-fat diet (around 10 percent calories from fat) is very practical or enjoyable. I have spent 15 years lightening recipes and suggesting alternatives in restaurants and supermarkets, so that people can easily enjoy a lower-fat way of life (around 20 to 30 percent calories from fat). So here we are with a recommendation to avoid eating a high-fat diet because it may help us prevent colon cancer. Over the recent years, I have altered my emphasis on food fat a little so that people are not only eating a moderate-fat diet, but are also switching to what are considered the more protective fats (monounsaturated fats—omega-9 fatty acids and omega-3 fatty acids) whenever possible.

One of the questions people often ask me is "What about butter?" I still use butter when it is truly the best fat for the recipe or dish. I just make a point of using less. The other question people ask me is "Which should I buy, canola oil or olive oil?" I answer, "both." Olive oil has phytochemicals (found in olives) that canola oil doesn't have, but canola oil contributes a plant form of omega-3 fatty acid. Canola oil has a neutral flavor and can be heated at high temperatures. Olive oil has a pleasant distinctive flavor that you want in only certain dishes. So, I use whichever oil compliments the dish best.

Evidence linking cancer of the colon with dietary fat was considered in several reports and studies to be stronger than the evidence linking dietary fat to breast cancer (National Research Council, 1989; Henderson et al., 1991).

A study was published in the April 1999 issue of *Carcinogenesis*. In it, rats were put on diets with low, medium, or high amounts of fat and either a fermentable fiber source (galacto-oligosaccharide), or a non-fermentable fiber source (cellulose), for nine months. Colorectal tumors were then induced with a chemical. Generally, the researchers found that the tumor incidence went up along with the fat content of the diet, and the fermentable GOS fiber offered greater protection against colorectal cancer than the diet with the non-fermentable cellulose (*Carcinogenesis*, vol. 20, No.4, 651-656, April, 1999).

Does the type of fat consumed relate to colon cancer prevention?

It's still under investigation, but it's looking like a yes. Some researchers believe that the association between total fat intake and cancer is stronger than the association between any specific type of fat and cancer.

So far, studies are starting to suggest a link between diets high in saturated fat and a risk of several types of cancer. Animal studies have shown that diets with a high saturated fat content are linked with increased numbers of intestinal bacteria (anaerobic, or non-oxygen), which are suspected of producing toxins or carcinogens that encourage polyp formation and enhance tumor progression (*Journal of the American Medical Association* August 2, 1995).

The 15 top total fat and saturated fat sources

We can't really begin to follow the food step to eat less saturated fat and avoid high-fat meals without knowing which foods are contributing the most fat and saturated fat to our diet. Focusing on the top 15 total fat and saturated fat sources seems like a great place to start. Luckily some nutritionists with the National Cancer Institute took a look at data from the USDA 1989-91 Continuing Survey of Food Intakes data, and ranked the top food sources of saturated fat in American adults. Here they are:

1. **Cheese (12.7 percent)**
   - Choose some of the reduced-fat cheeses.
   - When you eat or cook with cheese, use less.

2. **Beef (12.4 percent)**
   - Select the leaner cuts.
   - Trim off visible fat.
   - Eat beef less often.
   - Eat less beef when you do have it.

3. **Milk (10.5 percent)**
   - Use reduced-fat milk.
   - Take a look at how much you drink. Are you drinking enough water?

4. **Cakes/cookies/quick breads/doughnuts (5 percent)**
   - Make or buy them with a reduction in fat or saturated fat but only if you don't notice a difference in taste and they are truly satisfying!

5. **Margarine (4.8 percent)**
   - When you use margarine, try to use the absolute least amount possible.

- Buy a canola or olive oil tub margarine that has very few grams of saturated fat and trans fat.
- In recipes, use canola or olive oil instead of margarine whenever possible.

6. Butter (4.1 percent)

- Same as margarine.

7. Frozen yogurt (3.8 percent)

- There are some great tasting "light" ice creams out there.
- Check the label out to make sure it isn't just as high in calories and sugar as the regular version.

8. Salad dressings/mayo (3.7 percent)

- Make tasty reduced-fat salad dressings at home.
- Choose bottled salad dressings that use canola or olive oil and contain 5 to 7 grams fat per 2-tablespoon serving.
- When you use mayo, use less.
- Blend 1/3 Best Foods with 2/3 fat-free or "light" sour cream for a tasty but reduced-fat mayo blend.

9. Poultry (3.5 percent)

- Take off the skin before you cook the chicken whenever possible.
- Stick to lower-fat poultry choices and try not to have those deep fried chicken pieces and parts too often.

10. Other fats (3.4 percent)

- Same as oils below.

11. Oils (3.2 percent)

- Switch to canola or olive oil in your recipes.
- Use the least amount of oil you can get away with.

12. Sausage (2.8 percent)

- Switch to a reduced-fat sausage when possible.
- If an ingredient in a recipe, use less.
- Sausage is a "sometime" food.

13. **Yeast bread (2.7 percent)**

14. **Eggs (2.4 percent)**
    - When making a mostly egg dish, use half real eggs and half egg whites or egg substitute.

15. **Potato chips/corn chips/popcorn (2.3 percent)**
    - Potato chips are a "sometime" food. When you do have them, try not to eat the whole bag.
    - Choose the reduced-fat chips out there that you think taste great. Some even use canola oil.

(*Journal of the American Dietetic Association* 1998; 98:537-547.)

The heavy hitters

The big three saturated fat sources in the typical American diet are cheese, beef, and milk. Add in the next three heavy hitters—cakes/cookies, quick breads and doughnuts, margarine and butter (with margarine actually contributing .7 percent more saturated fat than butter)—and the top six sources total half of the saturated fat taken in on an average day in America.

The big four total fat sources are beef, margarine, salad dressing/mayonnaise, and cheese. Add these four up and they account for over a third of the total fat taken in each day. I've got to admit to being somewhat shocked by a few things on this list. Can you believe the salad dressings/mayonnaise grouping actually contributes more fat to the American diet than cheese? And that margarine accounts for almost 9 percent of the fat intake, with butter weighing in at a paltry 2.3 percent of the total fat? Adding up the first seven sources (beef, margarine, salad dressing/mayo, cheese, milk, cakes/cookies/quick breads/doughnuts, and poultry) not even including oils, totals half of the total fat in the typical American diet.

Here's my two cents

It sure looks like we should avoid excessive amounts of fat and saturated fat for other types of cancer, heart disease, and to reduce our risk of obesity. So if there is even a glimmer of evidence suggesting it can help reduce our risk of colon cancer, it deserves our attention.

We basically want to keep the trans fatty acids, saturated fat, and omega-6 fatty acids low. This leaves monounsaturated fats (olive oil and canola oil) and omega-3 fatty acids (fish, some plant foods, and canola oil) as our fats of choice. These are the fats that may be beneficial for our health in reasonable, moderate amounts.

But remember...it's not just about the fat

Eating less fat is only one step. All the other food steps to freedom fit together to form a healthier, leaner lifestyle. It isn't just about the type or the amount of fat. It's about eating more vegetables, fruits, fish, and whole grains, and eating less sugar and red meat and drinking less alcohol.

Cooking with less fat and saturated fat

I have a national column and a cookbook called *The Recipe Doctor*. My mission is to lighten up dishes and/or improve their nutritional attributes without sacrificing flavor, enjoyment, or free time. We're talking about real recipes for real people. You'll find tips on how to eat less fat and saturated fat when at restaurants in Chapter 8. Tips on shopping for less fat and saturated fat will be in Chapter 7.

I believe food is one of the great pleasures of life. I know what it's like to work hard and cook for a family of four. I don't want to spend hours in the kitchen—especially preparing "health" food that tastes mediocre. I'm figuring you don't either. So I don't peel, sift, whisk, or pull out the double boiler unless I absolutely have to. The point is that healthful food isn't going to do anyone any good if no one is eating it. The bottom line: It's got to taste great and it's got to be quick to make. Can it be done? You bet.

I don't believe in increasing the sugar or salt in a recipe to "get away with" using a lot less fat. And I don't believe there is a satisfactory substitute for chocolate or butter. So I still use them in certain recipes (when they are truly the best fats for the job), but I do use less.

I have found after lightening hundreds of recipes over the years that there is an ideal fat replacement and an ideal (smaller) amount of fat for almost every recipe. For example, if you cut the fat more than half in a cookie recipe, it isn't a cookie anymore—it's a muffin. Given my 15 or so years of recipe experimentation, I've learned a lot about lightening recipes. I have learned what works and what doesn't. I've assembled some of my lightening tricks below. Keep them handy and you'll be home free on this front.

Cooking tips to take home:

- When you cook or bake with less fat, you need to add other ingredients that help replace the qualities of the lost fat, while still adding flavors that complement the other ingredients in the original recipe.
- Start with the best tasting, freshest ingredients you can find. Fresh garlic, basil, and parsley, for example, have more flavor than if they are dried.
- Choose the best tasting "light" products on the market. For example, choose the creamiest "light" cream cheese and the sharpest reduced-fat cheese. Philadelphia light cream cheese, Cracker Barrel light sharp cheddar, Naturally Yours fat-free sour cream, and Louis Rich turkey bacon all taste terrific in recipes.
- Good nonstick cookware can help you cut the fat because it doesn't require as much to prevent sticking.
- Canola and olive oil cooking sprays help lubricate cookware and food, with a minimal amount of fat, by allowing you to spray tiny particles of fat onto the dish, pan, or food surface.
- Sometimes you can opt to use a cooking method that eliminates the need for cooking fat (broiling, roasting, poaching, or steaming).
- When fat is necessary to maintain the character of the food (oven frying, sautéing, pan frying, browning), do use it—just use less. Use canola or olive oil instead if you can.
- No additional fat is needed when using cake mixes. Most mixes already contain 4 grams of fat per serving of mix. Replace the oil called for with fruit juice, fruit puree, liqueur, flavored yogurt, chocolate syrup, or "light" sour cream, depending on the type of cake.

Ideal fat thresholds and fat replacements for different types of recipes

Recipe	Fat Threshold	Fat Replacements
Biscuits	4 tbs. shortening for every 2 cups flour.	Fat-free cream cheese, non-fat or "light" sour cream.
Cake mixes	No additional fat is needed because most mixes already have 4 grams of fat per serving; replace the oil that is called for with one of the fat replacements listed.	Non-fat or "light" sour cream, applesauce, pineapple juice, or liqueur, depending on the cake
Homemade cakes	1/4 to 1/3 cup shortening or butter per cake.	Liqueur for some cakes, coffee, "light" sour cream for chocolate ones; fruit juice or purees work well with carrot, apple, and spice cakes.
Cheese sauce	Omit butter; the cheese is the vital fatty ingredient; use a sharp, reduced-fat cheddar.	Make your thickening paste by mixing Wondra flour with a little bit of milk, then whisk in the remaining milk called for in the recipe.
Cookies	Generally you can only cut the fat by half. If the original recipe calls for 1 cup of butter, for example, try cutting it to 1/2 a cup.	Fat-free cream cheese for rich cookies; some fruit purees may work in fruit drop cookies. Maple syrup for oatmeal cookies.
Frosting		Cut the fat in half by using a high quality diet margarine, such as I Can't Believe It's Not Butter Light.
Marinades	1 tablespoon canola oil per cup of marinade (or none at all).	Fruit juices or beer to help balance the sharpness of the more acidic ingredients (vinegar, tomato juice).
Muffins and nut breads	2 tablespoons canola oil for a 12-muffin recipe.	Fat-free sour cream, flavored yogurts, fruit purees, maple syrup.

Ideal fat thresholds and fat replacements for different types of recipes (cont.)

Recipe	Fat Threshold	Fat Replacements
Pie and other pastry crusts	3 tablespoons shortening or canola margarine for every 1 cup flour.	Use fat-free cream cheese and substitute buttermilk for the required water.
Vinaigrette dressings	1 to 2 tablespoons olive or canola oil per 1/2 cup dressing.	Fruit juice, fruit purees (raspberry or pear), light corn syrup, maple syrup, non-alcoholic wines (depending on the recipe).
White sauces and gravies	1 teaspoon butter per serving of sauce.	Add a little more milk or broth to replace the lost fat. I use whole milk for a rich white sauce because, to me, whole milk is cream.

- In cookie recipes, you can cut the fat by a third or half. Fat-free cream cheese is one of the most successful fat replacements in cookie recipes—just blend it with the softened butter, shortening, or canola margarine, and proceed with the recipe. For example, if the cookie recipe calls for 1 cup of butter, blend 1/2 a cup with 1/2 a cup of fat-free cream cheese and continue on with the recipe.
- You can use diet margarine to make frosting. The water added should not be a problem if the frosting isn't heated and stays chilled.
- Use whole milk or the new fat-free half-and-half as a substitute for real half-and-half. It gives the recipe a richness and creaminess that you just can't get with non-fat or low-fat milk. If liquid whipping cream is called for, in order to end up with a great-tasting dish, you may need to use real half-and-half in its place.
- When you change the fat content of a batter or dough, you also change the way heat is conducted through the food. I found the best results (even heat distribution

and less burning) when using the Cushionaire bakeware line (the double thickness bakeware).

- There is something about the construction of corn syrup that makes it hold on to its moisture in a baked item longer. It actually seems to release its moisture slowly into the baked food. You can reduce the amount of granulated sugar called for in baking recipes (so the calories from sugar won't increase) and then replace some of the fat with corn syrup.

- Whipped egg whites can add a light texture to baked items. Egg whites whip best at room temperature. They must be separated from the yolk (egg yolks prevent the whites from holding air). Use a glass, copper, or stainless steel bowl for whipping egg whites (plastic tends to hold onto grease even after cleaning, and aluminum can react chemically with eggs and turn them grayish.) Don't over-beat your egg whites. They will collapse and separate. Stabilizing ingredients (like salt, lemon juice, and cream of tartar) help keep the whites smooth and aerated, but will also slow the whipping process, so add them just after the eggs become frothy.

- You can often reduce the number of egg yolks in a recipe simply because it can be done without visible ramifications. Egg yolks contain all the cholesterol in the egg, (about 200 milligrams apiece) and keeping cholesterol moderate still seems to be a good idea. But egg yolks also contain 5 grams of fat each. If it is an egg dish, such as quiche, omelet, frittata, or strata, it usually works wellto split the recipe evenly between real eggs egg substitute. So if the recipe calls for six eggs, use three eggs and 3/4 cup egg substitute.

Each recipe has an ideal fat threshold, the minimum amount of oil, butter, margarine, or shortening needed to produce a food that tastes like its fat-laden original. If you go below this ideal amount, and if you don't use a suitable fat replacement for the fat you've taken out, you won't be happy with the results. After years of lightening recipes for my column and cook-books, I've learned from my successes (and failures), and come up with the table on pages 60 and 61 listing ideal fat thresholds and fat replacements for different types of recipes.

Step 6: Keep extra weight minimal or off

Obesity and inactivity are generally considered to be among the most important risk factors for developing colorectal cancer by some experts. Being overweight has long been recognized as a risk factor for hormone related (and other) cancers (*European Journal of Cancer Prevention* 1999 Dec. 9 Suppl 1:S53-60).

A six-year study at the University of Pittsburgh found men with waists larger than 36 inches were twice as likely to develop colon cancer than thinner men. Researcher Robert Schoen, M.D. suspects that having fat around your belly is associated with increased insulin levels, which may be one of the things encouraging colon cancer to grow.

Italian studies found that excessive weight at certain ages predicts colorectal cancer risk in men, whereas how much weight is around the middle is a more reliable risk indicator for women. For more information on why fad diets are a waste of time, and for the latest research on shedding extra body fat for good, see Chapter 5.

Step 7: Eat several servings of whole grains a day

Whenever I use the word "several" in a sentence, my little girls always ask me, "how many is several again?" In my book, it means "about three." More than three is only going to give you more phytochemicals, fiber, vitamins, and minerals. But considering the average American currently eats less than one serving of whole grain each day, eating several a day is probably plenty challenging for now.

The good news about fiber

Lately, the link between high fiber diets and colon cancer prevention has been challenged by some surprising study results. Here's what the American Institute for Cancer Research makes of this:

"Although some studies on fiber and colorectal cancer have been inconclusive, many studies have shown that diets high in fiber and low in fat reduce colorectal cancer risk."

The proposed primarily plant-based diet with plenty of vegetables, fruits, beans, and whole grains gives us not only fiber, but also important vitamins, minerals, antioxidants, and other phytochemicals that help fight cancer.

And there is a lot more to fiber than just fighting colon cancer. A diet rich in soluble fiber can help the body in five big ways.

1. Lowers serum cholesterol and triglycerides.
2. Helps those with diabetes reduce their blood sugar and insulin levels and can lessen the chances of developing type 2 diabetes to begin with.
3. Helps people eat fewer calories by filling them up faster.
4. Helps the bowel by promoting general colon health by regulating bowel movements.
5. Helps lower blood pressure.

Soluble fiber forms a gel in the intestinal tract, which helps slow carbohydrate absorption, which in turn reduces the rise in blood glucose and insulin following the meal. Soluble fiber also grabs some bile as it is about to leave the body. The body then makes more bile—using cholesterol in the body—thereby reducing serum cholesterol levels.

All these body benefits can be yours with a higher fiber diet. The American Heart Association recommends people eat 25 to 30 grams of fiber from food, not supplements, each day. You'll find soluble fiber in beans, peas, oats, oat bran, barley, some fruits (such as apples, pears, prunes, berries, peaches, and citrus fruits), some vegetables (such as potatoes and sweet potatoes, parsnips and turnips, squash, broccoli, carrots, cauliflower, and asparagus), psyllium seed, and flaxseed.

- A study from the University of Texas Southwestern Medical Center in Dallas found that a high-fiber diet (including 25 grams each of soluble and insoluble fiber) relying on fruits, vegetables, and grains (not supplements), lowered blood sugar and insulin levels at least 10 percent more in type 2 diabetics than the standard American Diabetes Association diet with 24 grams of fiber a day.
- The same study from the University of Texas Southwestern Medical Center in Dallas noticed that for the group eating 50 grams of fiber a day, blood lipid levels (total cholesterol, triglycerides, and very low-density lipoproteins) decreased in amounts normally seen with lipid-lowering medications.
- With every 3-gram per day increase in soluble fiber, Finnish researchers (*Circulation* 1996; 94:2720-2727) found a 27 percent reduction in coronary death.
- Researchers at Northwestern University Medical School in Chicago found that adding oats (a great source of soluble fiber) to an already low-fat diet can help women lower cholesterol an additional 8 to 9 mg/dl. on top of the 12 mg/dl. reduction realized on the low-fat diet alone.
- Researchers from the department of epidemiology at Tulane University in New Orleans analyzed 19 years of data on what people ate in relationship to heart disease. They found that those who ate beans at least four times a week had a 19 percent lower risk for coronary disease.
- Research dietitians at Colorado State University gave a small group of men, ages 50 to 75, two bowls of high-fiber cereal (hot and cold oat and wheat cereals) every day for 12 weeks. They found that, on average, the amount of fat in their overall diets dropped from 91 grams a day to 82 grams. Saturated fat and cholesterol from food also dropped.
- Many studies have shown that a fiber-rich diet helps you stay (or get) trim by giving you a feeling of fullness and satiety after a meal sooner (so you are less

likely to overeat). It can help you feel this fullness longer (delaying the time when you feel physical hunger again).

Great news about whole grains

There are powerful nutrients and phytochemicals (plant chemicals) in whole grains that have recently been linked to reducing the risk of some cancers and heart disease. Here are the various phytochemicals whole grains contain and the health benefits they boast:

Lignans (barley, flaxseed)

Lignans function as antioxidants, which help prevent certain cellular changes that can lead to cancer. Studies have found that women with the highest concentrations of lignin in their urine are less likely to develop breast cancer than women with lower lignin levels.

Flavonoids (oats)

One of the flavonoids, rutin, may reduce heart disease risk by preventing platelets from clumping together. Rutin is also suspected of helping shrink LDL cholesterol particles and making them less likely to stick to arterial walls. Other flavonoids may reduce cell proliferation (rapid growth) and keep toxic substances from reaching cells.

Tocotrienols (whole wheat, oats, barley)

Tocotrienols are powerful antioxidants that help prevent ordinary LDL cholesterol from changing to a form that is especially likely to clog arteries. They also inhibit the production of cholesterol by the liver. And some saponins are thought to bind up cholesterol and usher it out of the body unabsorbed.

(**Note:** Whole grains also contribute vitamin E and selenium, which are both important antioxidants.)

•••

How phytochemicals work together with fiber, minerals, and vitamins is important. The only way to cover our bases here is to get all of these wonderful things together, in food. Many experts agree that making the effort to eat more whole grain foods is probably a better investment in your health than taking nutrition supplements.

In two recent studies with laboratory rats, whole wheat and rye came out on top. A higher wheat bran intake resulted in a decrease in intermediate biomarkers of colon carcinogenisis (*Journal of Parenteral Enteral Nutrition* 1999, Sept.-Oct. 23(5) 269-77). Rye bran supplementation decreased the frequency of colon cancer (*Carcinogenesis* 1999 June 20(6) 927-31).

What do we mean by whole grains?

There are at least nine varieties of cereals we can eat. When they are "whole" they have not been deprived of their bran and the germ portion of the grain. The grain is whole or intact.

- Wheat (whole wheat bread, cereals, and other whole wheat products).
- Oats.
- Barley.
- Rice (whole brown rice).
- Corn.
- Millet.
- Rye.
- Sorghum.
- Triticale.

The following are commonly referred to as grains but are botanically different. I've listed them here because they have similar nutritional attributes and are often prepared the same way as the other whole grains listed above.

- Buckwheat.
- Wild rice.
- Quinoa.
- Amaranth.
- Flaxseed.

Just eat one whole grain cereal a day

Just by eating one whole grain breakfast cereal every day, you get a list of health benefits a mile long. This is something many of us can definitely do—if not first thing in the morning as part of a complete breakfast, then later as an afternoon or bedtime snack. It's one of those great health habits to get used to doing on a daily basis. Here are some of the known benefits:

Helps reduce the risk of type 2 diabetes

Research from the Harvard School of Public Health and Brigham and Women's Hospital found that women who have a diet with a low intake of cereal fiber and a high sugar (glycemic) index diet have double the risk of type 2 diabetes (*Journal of the American Medical Association* 1997; 277: 472-477).

Helps reduce the risk of heart attack

Researchers studying the dietary intake and habits of male health professionals found that for every 10-gram increase in cereal fiber eaten each day, the risk of heart attack (myocardial infarction) was reduced by nearly 30 percent (*Journal of the American Medical Association* 1996: 275:447-451). A more recent study found this beneficial effect of cereal fiber is even stronger in women (*Journal of the American Medical Association,* June 2, 1999).

Helps reduce homocysteine levels in the blood, which helps reduce the risk of heart disease and other vascular disorders

Folic-acid-fortified breakfast cereals are very effective at reducing homocysteine blood concentrations (high levels of the amino acid homocysteine increase the risk of heart disease and other vascular disorders). After 12 weeks of eating folic-acid-fortified breakfast cereal as part of a low-fat diet, total homocysteine decreased by 24 percent (*American Journal of Clinical Nutrition* 2000; 71:1448-1454).

Helps reduce serum cholesterol

Researchers at Northwestern University Medical School in Chicago found that adding oats to an already low-fat diet helped women with serum cholesterol levels of above 200 mg/dl., lower cholesterol an additional 8 to 9 mg/dl after only three weeks. That's on top of the 12 mg/dl. reduction realized on the low-fat diet alone.

(Findings were presented by Linda Van Horn, Ph.D., R.D., at the First International Conference on Women, Heart Disease, and Stroke in Victoria, British Columbia, May, 2000.)

Helps reduce the risk of some cancers

A Swiss study found that whole grain cereals were protective for the oral cavity, pharynx, esophagus, and larynx cancer, compared to refined grains, which were associated with an increased risk of these cancers (*European Journal of Clinical Nutrition* 2000 June; 54(6): 487-489).

Helps reduce the amount of fat, saturated fat, and food cholesterol eaten throughout the day

In a recent study, men ate high fiber hot cereal for breakfast, and a serving for a snack (both oat and wheat cereals were used) for 12 weeks. In addition to increasing their daily fiber from an average of 19 grams a day to 30 grams a day, the men experienced an unintentional 10 percent drop in grams of fat eaten. Grams of saturated fat and dietary cholesterol also dropped. (Data presented on June 5, 2000, by Brenda Davy, R.D., research dietitian, Colorado State University, Fort Collins, at the American Heart Association conference on cardiovascular health in Reston, Va.)

For a list of whole grain breakfast cereals, check out Chapter 7. For a few recipes using whole grain breakfast cereals, check out Chapter 6.

Tips to take home:

- Start the day with a whole grain cereal that contains at least 5 grams of fiber per serving. Top with wheat germ, flaxseed, raisins, bananas, or berries (or a combination). These all add fiber and other nutrients.
- If you don't like cereal for breakfast, or you have a day when you happen to have something else first thing in the morning, have your whole grain cereal with low-fat milk later in the day as an afternoon or bedtime snack.
- Make a yogurt parfait in a tall glass, alternating layers of fresh fruit, whole grain cereal (Grape Nuts and granola work well here), and your favorite flavor of yogurt.

- Start collecting recipes for wonderful tasting whole grain muffins (there are two in the recipe chapter of this book). Muffins are a great breakfast or snack. Just make a batch, wrap them individually, and throw them in the freezer. When you want one, just microwave for 30 to 60 seconds. If you want to grab it on your way out to work, it will be nicely thawed by mid-morning.
- Find whole grain bread that you like and start using it for toast and sandwiches.
- Look for healthful recipes that call for oats. You see oats in muffins, bread, granola, hot cereal, cookie, and bar recipes.
- Experiment with some of the less common whole grains, like barley. Look for recipes that call for barley (soups, casseroles, salads).
- There is nothing better than homemade bread fresh out of the oven. If you have a bread machine or like to make bread at home, find a whole grain bread or roll recipe you really like—even if it used half white flour and half whole wheat flour, at least you are getting some whole grain.

Step 8: Take a multivitamin containing some folic acid, calcium, and vitamin E

Although you can (and should) get most of the vitamins and minerals you need through food sources, the reality is that most of us don't. Many of us end up taking a vitamin-mineral supplement to help make up the balance—as a nutrition insurance policy. Most health professionals agree vitamin supplements are not a substitute for a healthy diet and lifestyle. In other words, a vitamin pill isn't going to make a high-fat diet any lower in fat or a low-fiber diet any higher in fiber.

But lately we are seeing research popping up that is finding some health benefits to taking a multivitamin a day—even for colon cancer risk reduction....

Focusing on folate (folic acid)

A new study from the researchers at Harvard Medical School suggests that folate (folic acid) supplementation is effective in preventing colon cancer. They found that the women who took a multivitamin containing a folate supplement for 15 or more years had a 75 percent reduced risk of colon cancer. Women who had been taking more than 400 mcg a day of folate showed a reduced risk of colon cancer, years later compared to those who took 200 mcg or less (*Patient Care*, Dec. 15, 1998 v32).

The findings were controlled for age, family history of colon cancer, aspirin use, smoking, body mass, physical activity, consumption of red meat, alcohol, the amino acid methionine, and fiber, as well as other components of multivitamins; vitamins A, C, D, E, and calcium. But only after 15 years of supplement use did the risk reduction become significant. This tells us that folate may help prevent the progression of these tumors in its early stages but probably does little to nothing for the more advanced tumors.

This means if a woman wants to have this benefit at the age of 50 to 60, when colon cancer risk kicks into high gear, she would have had to start taking the supplement 15 years sooner—at age 35.

How might it help? Some researchers speculate that the antioxidant-like folate keeps cells in the colon wall from mutating and growing out of control. Folate is called a methyl donor. It gives up a piece of its chemical structure, methyl, in order to discourage wayward cell growth.

Folic acid in food

Folic acid is added to breads and grain products, but you'll find it naturally in beans, dark green vegetables, and citrus fruits. Find out which plant foods are richest in folic acid. Take a look at the following list and circle the ones you like. You can make a point of choosing these power plant foods whenever possible. The following are the top 30 plant-based foods that contain folic acid:

1. Lentils (1/2 cup), 179 mcg.
2. Black beans, cooked (1/2 cup), 128 mcg.
3. Black-eyed peas, cooked (1/2 cup), 120 mcg.
4. Kidney beans, cooked (1/2 cup), 115 mcg.
5. Spinach, cooked (1/2 cup), 103 mcg.
6. Green soybeans, cooked (1/2 cup), 100 mcg.
7. Collard greens, cooked (1/2 cup), 88 mcg.
8. Asparagus spears (4), 84 mcg.
9. Navy beans, cooked (1/2 cup), 81 mcg.
10. Romaine lettuce (1 cup), 76 mcg.
11. Orange juice, fresh (1 cup), 75 mcg.
12. Pinto beans, canned (1/2 cup) 72 mcg.
13. Beets, cooked (1/2 cup), 68 mcg.
14. Brussels sprouts, cooked (1/2 cup), 67 mcg.
15. Split peas, cooked (1/2 cup), 64 mcg.
16. Spinach, fresh, chopped (1 cup), 58 mcg.
17. Tofu (1/2 cup), 55 mcg.
18. Papaya cubes (1 cup) 53 mcg.
19. Broccoli, cooked, chopped (1/2 cup), 52 mcg.
20. Mustard greens, cooked (1/2 cup), 51 mcg.
21. Vegetable-tomato juice (1 cup), 51 mcg.
22. Wheat germ (2 tablespoons) 50 mcg.
23. Green peas, cooked (1/2 cup), 47 mcg.
24. Artichoke hearts (1/2 cup), 43 mcg.
25. Okra, cooked (1/2 cup), 36 mcg.
26. Banana (1), 35 mcg.
27. Iceberg lettuce (1 cup), 31 mcg.
28. Orange (1 small), 29 mcg.
29. Mango (1 medium), 29 mcg.
30. Kiwi (1), 29 mcg.

The calcium connection

The best sources of calcium are milk and milk products. This has been drilled into our heads by dairy commercials throughout our lives. We are supposed to get more calcium as we age in order to help preserve our bones. Now we are hearing that calcium could also be connected to all types of other health matters—from helping to lower high blood pressure to helping lower risk of colon cancer.

In a recent study, calcium supplementation (1200 milligrams a day for four years) lowered risk of colon cancer recurrence (in people with a history of colorectal cancer) by about 9 percent. Those people taking calcium supplements who had a recurrence had fewer tumors than those not taking the calcium supplement (*New England Journal of Medicine*, Jan 14, 1999 vol. 340).

Preliminary evidence suggests that taking calcium supplements or increasing dietary calcium intake reduces colon cancer risk by inhibiting cell proliferation on the walls of the colon (*Harvard Health Letter*, Nov 1, 1998 vol. 24).

Certainly, more needs to be known on calcium and colon cancer, but why not make an extra point of getting the recommended daily intake of calcium, as we need to for our bones and blood pressure anyway. The list below will help get you well on your way to higher calcium intake.

You may think it will be difficult to get a good amount of calcium in your diet. After all, there's a big jump from the amount of calcium in a cup of broccoli, (84 mg) to the amount in a cup of yogurt (448 mg). But it all adds up. A cup of yogurt here, a cup of broccoli there, an ounce of cheese, and a cup of kale later and suddenly, you're almost at 1,000 mg! Here are the top 24 calcium-rich foods:

1. Low-fat yogurt (1 cup), 448 mg.
2. Blackstrap molasses (2 tablespoons), 350 mg.
3. Cottage cheese (1 cup), 306 mg.
4. Non-fat milk (1 cup), 300 mg.
5. Whole milk (1 cup), 290 mg.
6. Spinach, cooked (1 cup), 280 mg.
7. Sardines with bones (3.5 ounces), 240 to 380 mg.
8. Cheese, reduced-fat (1 ounce), 207 mg.
9. Cheese, whole milk (1 ounce), 204 to 272 mg.
10. Collard greens, cooked (1 cup), 200 mg.
11. Beet greens, cooked (1 cup), 164 mg.
12. Tofu (1/2 cup), 138 mg.
13. Green soybeans, cooked (1/2 cup), 130 mg.
14. Soy nuts, roasted (1/2 cup), 119 mg.
15. Mustard greens, cooked (1 cup), 102 mg.
16. Swiss chard, cooked (1 cup), 102 mg.

17. Butternut squash, cooked (1 cup), 100 mg.
18. Okra, cooked (1 cup), 100 mg.
19. Kale, cooked (1 cup), 94 mg.
20. Ice cream, vanilla (1/2 cup), 85 mg.
21. Broccoli, cooked (1 cup), 84 mg.
22. Navy/baked beans (1/2 cup), 64 mg.
23. Artichoke, cooked (1 whole), 54 mg.
24. Pinto beans, canned (1/2 cup), 52 mg.

Vitamin E

Women who took in 66 IU of vitamin E a day (twice the recommended daily allowance) reduced their risk for colon cancer by 68 percent, compared to women who consumed the recommended amount of vitamin E. (These results are from a five-year study of 32,215 women presented at the 1993 annual conference of the American Society of Preventive Oncology.) The association between vitamin E and a reduced risk of colon cancer appears to taper off in women over age 65.

We know that vitamin E has a strong ability to protect cell membranes against destruction. Keeping cell membranes strong could be particularly important in the colon because the bacteria in the colon produce a lot of free radicals.

Watch out for iron

If you have reached menopause, you should choose from the low-iron multivitamin supplements out there. If you've stopped having your period prematurely (from a hysterectomy, for example), you should be taking the "silver" or "senior" type multivitamins because they tend to be the ones with the lowest amounts of iron. (For more on this see "Ironing out Your Red Meat" in step 4.)

How to choose the right supplement

If you are going to take something every day for years and years, it pays to do the math and label reading to find the best supplement possible from the beginning. By "best," I mean a supplement that is:

Complete

Nutrients work together, so it is best to choose a supplement that includes a complete mix of all the vitamins and minerals with established RDAs:

- The B vitamins (Thiamin, Riboflavin, Niacin, B-6, folate (folic acid), B-12, Biotin, and Pantothenic acid).
- Vitamin A.
- Vitamin C.
- Vitamin D.
- Vitamin E.
- Calcium.
- Copper.
- Iodine.
- Iron.
- Magnesium.
- Phosphorus.
- Zinc.

You also might consider making sure it contains chromium, as it is one of the minerals we might need more of as we age. (There isn't an RDA established for chromium so you might want to check if your supplement contains the minimum amount [50 micrograms] suggested by the RDA committee.)

Balanced

Read the nutrition label for the supplement and make sure it provides close to 100 percent of the RDA for most of the vitamins and minerals. With that said, you'll find that biotin isn't usually present at this level because it is particularly expensive. Calcium and magnesium aren't at the 100 percent mark because they are so bulky. If they were included, the pills would be too large to swallow.

You don't want to get too much more than 100 percent of the RDA for these vitamins and minerals. Many can cause medical problems (or discomfort) in excessive doses. High doses can also negatively effect the benefits of others. Unless you have a specific reason for doing so, and know it's safe, it's best to avoid more than 100 percent of any vitamins and minerals (except perhaps vitamin E) in supplement form.

Contains calcium but not too much iron

The amounts of calcium in the supplements listed below range from 13 to 60 percent of the RDA (most provide 16 percent).

Supplements that contain more than 100 percent of the RDA for iron were left out of the list. Ten percent of the population is genetically prone to iron overload. There is also that possible link between excessive iron and colon cancer.

Takes no longer than 30 minutes to disintegrate

In order for your body to be able to absorb and use the vitamins and minerals in your supplement, the pill must first dissolve while it is in your stomach or small intestine. If it takes longer than 30 minutes to dissolve, the tablet will probably pass through you and end up supplementing your sewer system instead. All the supplements below meet the disintegration standards proposed by U.S. Pharmacopeia (USP), the scientific organization that establishes drug standards. Such supplements disintegrate completely within 30 to 45 minutes.

Tips to take home:

- Don't buy a supplement that is close to (or past) its expiration date. Vitamins are sensitive to heat and air and can lose their potency over time.
- Some supplements include botanical substances in addition to vitamins and minerals. Remember: if you take a botanical supplement, do so at your own risk. There are known risks involved with taking too much of some herbal supplements. Consult your doctor or nurse practitioner before considering a botanical or herbal supplement.
- Don't take supplements on an empty stomach. Take your supplements with or after a meal, when they have a better chance of being dissolved and absorbed. This is partly because many of the vitamins and minerals are more likely to be absorbed in the presence of other nutrients. (Calcium is absorbed in the presence of vitamin D and magnesium.)
- Talk with your health care provider. To avoid unwanted interactions with other medications, tell your doctor or nurse practitioner about all the supplements you take. Certain medications might make your supplements useless, or vice-versa.

A few good supplements

Brand	$ per mo.	Folate	Calcium	Iron
		(—— percent RDA ——)		
Centrum Silver*	$3.50	100%	20%	22%
Centrum	$3.50	100%	16%	100%
One-A-Day Maximum	$3.85	100%	13%	100%

* Centrum Silver contains 150 percent of the RDA for vitamin E, (45 IU) whereas the regular version contains 100 percent. Centrum Silver also contains 416 percent of the RDA for B-12 and 150 percent RDA for B-6, whereas the regular version contains 100 percent.

- No matter what, food must still come first on your list of nutritional priorities. Nature made it complete and balanced. We have yet to discover enough about all the phytochemicals and other beneficial substances in foods to be able to reproduce them in pill form. We don't know all there is to know about how nutrients work with one another to prevent disease. The safest and most economical bet is food in its whole, unprocessed (or minimally processed) form.

Step 9: Do not overdo sugary foods and alcohol

Avoiding sugar makes it into the 10 food steps to freedom because it may be linked to obesity. Obesity is linked to colon cancer on its own merit, which is why keeping off extra weight has its very own food step (food step 6). Not overdoing sugary foods includes avoiding soft drinks, sweetened coffee and fruit drinks, cakes, cookies, candy, sweetened cereals, and so on. A recent review of international research on this topic concluded that a high fat intake is the most important single cause for obesity, but that a high sugar intake could not be excluded as a contributing factor. For most people, the best advice would be not only to look at trimming extra sugar calories but also to eat a variety of foods in reasonable portion sizes along with at least 30 minutes of exercise every day.

It's not that sugar is "bad"

It's not that sugar is "bad"...it just isn't good for you in excessive amounts. Excessive amounts are what the typical American gets. Soda and fruit drinks, candy, chocolate, ice cream, and cookies are leading the pack.

The science linking sugar to colon cancer

There are studies that find a correlation between a high-sugar diet and colorectal cancer, and studies that don't. But one of the most recent and largest studies on women found sugar-filled foods and drinks, along with sugar intake, to be risk factors for colon cancer (*Cancer Causes and Control*, 1994, 5, 38-52). Several animal studies have shown that replacing sugar with starch protects rats against colorectal cancer (*Journal of Nutrition* 123, 704-712, and *Journal of Nutrition* 124, 517-523).

An Italian study looked at intake of refined bread and sugar and found that people with the highest intake of refined bread had a 28 percent higher risk of colorectal cancer than those with the lowest intake had. An increase of one serving (4 teaspoons) of refined sugar per day showed an 11 percent increase in colorectal cancer risk (*European Journal of Cancer Prevention* 7 [Supp 2]: S19-S23).

The association between high-sugar diets and colon cancer isn't as far-fetched as it sounds. A high-sugar diet does appear to increase the time food waste stays in the colon (colon transit time). It also increases the concentration of bile acids in feces (*Gut*, 1991, 32, 367-371). Both of these are thought to increase the risk of colon cancer. We also don't know whether the sugar itself promotes cancer, or whether sugar replaces cancer-protective foods that help prevent the cancer. A high-sugar diet might be linked to an increased risk of colon cancer, but more studies need to be done before we know for sure.

We are eating more sugar than ever before

We are eating more sugar than ever before—20 teaspoons' worth of added sugars every day, according to the USDA's 10th nationwide food consumption survey (1994 to 1996). That's 20 percent more sugar than we consumed in 1986. And the 20 teaspoons doesn't even include sugars found naturally in foods like fruits and milk. That's about 320 calories (16 percent of the total calories for adults).

The American Dietetic Association recently advised consumers to enjoy sugars in moderation as part of a healthful diet. The problem is, many of us aren't eating healthful diets to begin with, and at an average of 20 teaspoons of sugar a day, we're not exactly moderating our sugar intake either. The higher the portion of our calories from sugar, the harder it is to eat a healthful diet and meet our nutrient needs.

How much sugar is recommended?

The USDA recommends we get no more than 6 to 10 percent of our total calories from added sugar (that's about six teaspoons per 1,600 calories).

The fat factor

Fat is one aspect of some of our favorite high-sugar foods that can put us in double jeopardy. Ice cream, chocolate, and other rich sweets are just as high in extra fat as they are in sugar. The higher the fat and sugar, the higher the calories, and the more likely those extra calories will contribute to weight gain.

Looking to trim some calories off your daily total? Start with sugar

By cutting daily sugar from 20 to eight teaspoons of sugar, you trim off 12 teaspoons of sugar a day, or 180 extra calories. This computes to a savings of 5400 calories a month; a potential loss of 1 1/2 pounds of body fat a month. Let's do the math:

- 1 teaspoon of sugar = 15 calories.
- 12 less teaspoons of sugar a day x 15 calories each = 180 calories a day.
- 180 calories a day x 30 days = 5,400 calories saved a month.
- 1 pound of body fat = 3,500 calories.
- 5,400 calories of saved calories ÷ 3,500 = 1 1/2 pounds.
- Over a year's time: 1 1/2 pounds of body fat lost per month x 12 months = 18 pounds per year!

Natural vs. refined sugar: Does your body know the difference?

Refined sugar and other sweeteners are mostly made up of what we call "empty" calories. This means you get calories without getting much of anything else. The calories from natural sugar in foods like fruits, milk, and beans come with fiber and a host of nutrients and phytochemicals. Does your body know the difference? This seems to depend on who you ask.

Several studies have shown that (as part of a high-carbohydrate, low-fat diet) insulin and triglyceride levels rose higher when a higher proportion of carbohydrates came from refined sugars, rather than carbohydrate plant foods like grains and produce. (Gerald Reaven, Stanford University, *Journal of Clinical Endocrinology Metabolism* 59: 636m 1984, and Christopher Gardner et al., Stanford University, *Canadian Journal of Cardiology* 13 [Suppl. B]: 236B, 1997.) There is no scientific agreement on how much added sugar, compared to naturally occurring sugar, is considered free from health risk.

Tips for enjoying sugars in moderation

When it comes to sugar, it's all about moderation. A little is great. A lot can get you into calorie overload. In other words, you can have your cake and eat it too—as long as the piece of cake is a sliver instead of a monster slice. Here are some tips that will hopefully help keep sugar moderate in your home.

- Most of the time you can add about 1/4 to 1/3 less sugar than the recipe calls for in muffins, cakes, cookies, pies and so on, without even noticing a difference in taste and texture.
- Only choose whole grain breakfast cereals that are lightly sweetened or have no sugar added. Avoid the heavily sugared cereals.
- Dessert servings can be shared with friends or family when at restaurants.
- Eliminate fruits with added sugars. Buy unsweetened frozen fruit and fruits canned in their own juices instead.
- Remember to choose water as your beverage whenever possible. Limit high calorie soft drinks, fruit drinks, and sweetened coffee and tea beverages to just one a day.
- Always reach for some fruit when your sweet tooth is calling. This will only work if it's a fruit you truly enjoy.
- Think portion control. Remember to look for serving sizes on food labels.
- If you don't mind the taste of artificial sweeteners, you haven't noticed any side effects from NutraSweet, and you've just got to have your soda, make it a diet soda, and keep it to one a day.
- Observe whether your energy level is more stable (and you are less likely to go for a quick-fix sugar rush) if you eat many mini-meals throughout the day, rather than skipping meals and eating one or two large ones.
- Never say never. If you try to cut sugar completely from your diet, you will most likely feel deprived and only want it more. Sugar isn't "bad." It's the amount of sugar and extra calories we are eating that we can cut back on. After all, we were born with a natural taste for sweetness.

Now, about alcohol

Alcohol is associated with a higher risk of colorectal cancers. The more you drink, the higher your colorectal cancer risk. It doesn't matter which type of alcohol you drink. Alcohol may inhibit the body's absorption of vitamins and minerals such as iron, zinc, vitamin E, and folate (the last two of which are potential cancer fighters), and alcohol may inhibit cells from being able to repair themselves. If you do drink, do so in moderation:

- One drink a day for women.
- Two drinks for men.
- Researchers advise that if you enjoy alcohol, limit yourself to three drinks a week.

Other reasons to drink in moderation

Keep in mind that results of six international studies estimated that drinking two to five alcoholic drinks a day raises a woman's risk of getting breast cancer by more than 40 percent. Thinking positively, if you keep alcohol within recommended limits, experts estimate it will help prevent up to 20 percent of cancers of the aerodigestive tract, the colon, rectum, and breast (*Food, Nutrition and the Prevention of Cancer: A Global Perspective,* 1997, American Institute for Cancer Research).

Five glasses of water every day

Here's something we should all be doing anyway. We hear it all the time—drink eight glasses of water a day. Women who drank more than five glasses of water each day (in a study at the Fred Hutchinson Cancer Research Center in Seattle), had a 50 percent less chance of developing colon cancer than women who drank fewer than two glasses of water each day. Men showed a small reduction in risk.

How is it helping? Water helps prevent constipation and speeds up the intestines in general (which might reduce the contact with, and concentrations of, carcinogens in the colon).

How can you drink more water? Here are some ideas:

- Drink water with every meal.
- Remember to rehydrate yourself mid-morning and mid-afternoon.

- Keep a fresh pitcher in the fridge so cold water is only a quick pour away.
- Take a water bottle of ice water with you when you're driving around. Sometimes this is the only time we have to sip some water.

Tips to take home:

Instead of having an alcoholic drink at the end of the day, at a restaurant, or at a party, you can:

- Order a fancy drink without the alcohol, such as a virgin daiquiri, margarita, or Bloody Mary.
- Enjoy many of the great tasting non-alcoholic beers and wines that are now available.
- Have a fancy coffee drink (without the alcohol).
- Ask the bartender for club soda or sparkling mineral water with a wedge of lemon or lime.
- Enjoy an iced or hot tea, or a glass of lemonade.
- Order hot chocolate, especially during the winter.
- If you are really thirsty, go for water, the ultimate thirst quencher.
- If you are finding it difficult to drink less or go a day without alcohol, please consider getting some medical advice or professional help.

Food Step 10: Stay active and exercise as much as possible

Exercise helps speed the passage of stools through the intestines. The other bonus to exercise is helping reduce excess weight, which is food step 6. Exercise is thought to boost metabolism (increasing the amount of calories we burn just maintaining our bodies), in addition to burning the calories we need to fuel our exercise.

Since 1980, seven out of eight studies that examined the relationship between physical activity and colon cancer concluded that exercise reduces the risk. These studies included people in significantly large numbers on several continents (North America, Europe, and Asia).

Just 30 minutes of walking a day cut colon cancer risk by 10 percent in the Harvard nurses' study. The walking sped up the time it took a stool to travel out of the intestine.

One large American study in 1984 found that men with sedentary occupations (such as accountants or lawyers) had a colon cancer risk 60 percent higher than men whose work required some exercise (such as carpenters or mail carriers). A similar Swedish study found that a sedentary job was associated with a 30 percent increase in cancer risk. Part of the decrease in risk as job-related exercise increases could also be due to other health habits. More studies will be needed to prove that exercise exerts an independent protective effect. (*Harvard Health Letter*, March 1992 vol. 17 n5 p5 [3]).

Today, most of us have sedentary jobs that keep us on our duff, which means unless we make a point to get some exercise in our off hours, our risk of colon cancer could increase by 30 percent or more.

If you haven't been exercising on a regular basis, getting started is the hardest part. Once you get going, and you start feeling the difference (more energy, better sleep), it's easier to keep it up. If you are a self-proclaimed couch potato, then maybe riding a stationary bike while you watch television is a good place to start.

Keys to exercise success

You are more likely to start exercising, and stay exercising, if you:
- See that there is a big benefit to doing it.
- Choose activities you actually enjoy.
- Feel comfortable and competent doing the activity.
- Feel safe doing the activity.
- Can get to the activity easily on a regular basis.
- Can fit the activity into your daily schedule.
- Feel that the exercise doesn't cost too much of your money or time.

- Incorporate these tips to be more active in your daily life:
    - Take the stairs.
    - Walk to lunch.
    - Get up to change the TV channel.
    - Garden.
    - Walk the dog.
    - Walk between stores instead of driving.

In one recent study (*Journal of the American Medical Association* 282:1554-60, 1999) researchers looked at which exercise group was able to maintain the most weight loss over an 18-month period. The group that exercised for short bouts (four to 10 minutes each time, totaling 40 minutes a day) gained the most weight back, and the group exercising for long bouts (five times a week, 40 minutes each time) gained back less weight than the first group. The group that maintained the most weight loss was the group that received treadmills for their homes. Having the equipment at home made it easier and more convenient for them to exercise on a regular basis.

Tips to take home:

- Find something you enjoy and you're more likely to stick to it.
- Discover what time of day you are most likely to exercise. For me this is late at night, after my entire family is in bed. I turn on the television, get on my stationary bike, and pedal away the day's stresses and frustrations, while I watch one of my favorite shows.
- Maybe you need more social types of exercise, such as dance classes or a walk with a neighbor, co-worker, or friend. When you are walking and talking with someone you really like, time flies by.
- Make a rainy day plan. Don't let the weather put a damper on your fitness schedule. Some people like to use exercise videos for this type of situation. Home exercise equipment comes in handy for this as well.

- Exercise in short spurts throughout the day. If you work in an office, walk from your car or subway, then take the stairs a few times during the day. Then do a little extra exercise at home in the evening.

It's important to speak with your doctor before beginning an exercise program or increasing the amount or intensity of the exercise you currently do.

Looking to future research

Researchers are looking into whether the following factors may help decrease colorectal cancer risk:

- Low-fat dairy products. (Various studies have suggested a link between low-fat dairy products and a diet adequate in calcium, with a lower risk of colon cancer, or lower recurrence of colorectal polyps. Calcium is thought to possibly inhibit damage in the colon from bile acids, which might encourage cancerous tumors.)
- Garlic.
- Calcium.
- Vitamins C, D, and E.
- Coffee.
- Regular use of aspirin. (The benefits of taking a single aspirin, 325 mg, four to six times a week, are being investigated.)
- Hormone replacement therapy in postmenopausal women.

Getting the motivation and know-how to follow the steps

Most of us are quite aware that we should be eating less red meat, saturated fat, and calories. We know we should be eating more fruits, vegetables, beans, whole grains, and fish, and exercising more. The truth is, knowing we should be doing it, and actually doing it, are two very different things.

What does it take to make these changes? Remember the four main stages in accepting loss—denial, anger, grief, acceptance. In a similar way, change doesn't come easily. However, there are stages of change too. Gradually, people become more focused on the disadvantages of the old behavior and the advantages of change. All of this takes time. Willpower is an essential ingredient for change, but willpower or commitment alone aren't enough. Many experts believe you need to prepare for change. These are the stages of change posited by psychologist James Prochaska:

1. **Precontemplation.** You have no current intention of changing. You might even feel a situation is hopeless. You use denial and defensiveness to keep from going forward. Raising consciousness may help move you forward at this stage.

2. **Contemplation.** You accept or realize you have a problem and you seriously think about changing it. A lot of people get stuck at this stage. They might be waiting for absolute certainty (which rarely exists), or they might be secretly hoping for another way out without having to change their behavior.

3. **Preparation.** You are starting to pull yourself in a new direction. You plan to take action within a month. You are starting to think more about the future than you think about the past. You think more about the positives of the new behavior than about the negatives of the old one. Telling others about your intentions and developing a plan for action can help at this stage.

4. **Action.** You start the new behavior. Rewarding yourself and making your environment as change-friendly as possible helps at this stage.

5. **Maintenance.** You are sticking with your new behavior. Remind yourself that maintenance is an ongoing process that is often more difficult to achieve than the action stage. Three things often prohibit maintenance: overconfidence, temptation, and blaming yourself for lapses. Expect these three common challenges to maintenance. In terms of relapses, just accept that there

will be some. Plan to learn from each relapse. Have a plan to help avoid or minimize the daily temptations you may have in your life. Keep going with your strategies for the action stage (commitment, reward, change-friendly environments, surrounding yourself with people who help and support your change, and so forth).

(James Prochaska, Ph.D., a psychologist and head of Health Promotion Partnership at the University of Rhode Island and author of *Changing for Good* [William Morrow and Company, 1994]).

That "M" word: Motivation

According to Dr. Prochaska, there are two ways to get more motivated: You can make a single motive extremely important, and/or increase the number of motives. That's what trying to prevent colon cancer does for many of us. It increases the number of motives. Surrounding ourselves with people who believe in and applaud our changes adds some motivation.

In order to help you prepare, take action, and maintain these healthful diet changes, you will find practical tips and information in the next four chapters. See Chapter 5 for practical advice on losing extra body fat, Chapter 6 for recipes, Chapter 7 for practical supermarket advice, and Chapter 8 for the do's and don'ts of take out and dining out.

 <u>Chapter 5</u>

Focus on Health...
Not Pounds

Eat and exercise for the health of it and let the pounds fall where they may

I don't believe in fad dieting. I feel it's simply one of the worst routes a person can take. The weight loss never lasts. Generally there is only a 5 percent success rate when you look at maintained weight loss over a five-year period. That means for every 100 people on these various diets, only five people—at best—haven't gained the weight back. Not only that, but anytime you embark in a quick weight loss scheme, you are making it more difficult for your body to shed pounds in the future. Each time you lose weight quickly, your body gets better and better at gaining it back and holding onto this extra weight the next time around. One of the reasons for this is because when you lose weight quickly, you tend to lose muscle mass and protein mass. But when the pounds come back on, they tend to come back as body fat. This loss in muscle decreases the amount of calories you burn just maintaining your basic body functions. The fewer calories you burn by maintaining your body's functions, the more likely you will have extra calories floating around after meals and put on extra body weight.

No one can go on these fad diets for very long because you eventually get tired of it. Anytime you are dieting, you are spending the bulk of your waking time and energy thinking about and following this new diet. Eating should be about satisfying hunger, nourishing your body, and enjoying the meal.

Maintaining the joy of eating

Healthful food isn't going to do anyone any good if no one's eating it. Food should be enjoyed. With all this talk about what's bad or good for our bodies, that enjoyment part can get lost in the

---

F.Y.I. Quick weight loss: What are you really losing?

You know the books and magazine articles claiming to help you "lose five pounds in five days?" When you lose five pounds in five days, you lose mostly water. Let me show you what you are really losing in the first few days.

Days 1-3 of a quick weight loss diet
- 75 percent of the weight loss is water.
- 20 percent of the weight loss is fat.
- 5 percent of the weight loss is protein.

Days 11-13
- 69 percent of the weight loss is fat.
- 19 percent of the weight loss is water.
- 12 percent of the weight loss is protein.

Days 21-24
- 85 percent of the weight loss is fat.
- 15 percent of the weight loss is protein.
- 0 percent of the weight loss is water.

nutritional shuffle. I don't feel this should happen. Because if it doesn't taste good, chances are, you won't be able to stick to your new healthful diet for very long.

There is something less obvious that can zap the joy right out of eating—counting. Counting calories, fat grams, or tabulating food group servings—take your pick. If you have to count any-thing having to do with your food, it will take the joy not only out of eating, but out of living. Anytime you put yourself in a count-ing mode, day in and day out, you automatically snap into the dieting mentality, which often leaves you feeling defeated, deprived, and depressed.

I don't mind periodic counting, when, every now and then, you check in to see how your average daily food intake compares to certain standards or recommendations. It can be useful as long as it is a checkpoint and not a daily regimen. There are people who, for their continued health, have to count certain nutrients (people with diabetes or renal disease). Believe me, one of their greatest challenges is maintaining the joy of eating.

Beauty is in the eye of the beholder

In some parts of the world and in other points in history, my curvy and round size 14 figure would be considered very desir-able. It was not until the early 1900s that the Rubenesque women painted by Rafael and Renoir (around the mid to late 1800s) were no longer considered the female ideal. In their time, extra weight on women was a sign of being rich and healthy.

It was in the early 1900s that corsets and the age of the thin flapper dancer became popular. In the mid-1900s, curves seemed to be coming back in with Marilyn Monroe (a gorgeous and curvy size 14), leading the charge. Unfortunately, today many women are now embarrassed to be a size 14.

The 1960s ushered in the age of miniskirts and bony women. I don't think we've shaken this yet, even after 30 plus years. Beauty contestants, models, and Hollywood actresses have never been thinner. Ironically, obesity and eating disorders in this coun-try have only been increasing. As a nation, in the past 20 years we have dumped billions of dollars into the dieting business. It hasn't worked. We've never been more unhappy and more obese. Why do we keep pumping more dollars into fad diets? Why aren't we pumping iron instead? Why do we hate our bodies? Why aren't we celebrating our curves and focusing on health and fitness instead?

Call me an optimist, but I think the pendulum is beginning to swing back a bit. Finally, there are more normal sized women models, thanks to Emme, and talk show host Rosie O'Donnell. There are starting to be truly fashionable clothing stores and catalogs for women size 12/14 on up. It's like a breath of fresh air. I have recently noticed television specials about larger sized women being the "new" idea of beauty (which is really an old idea that is just coming back).

Just the other night I was watching a cable special on what men and women (past and present) are looking for in a mate. The producers interviewed men and women in parts of northeastern Africa and the men in this particular village said they were looking for a wife who was strong, had wide hips, and could have many children. I remember thinking, hey, they're describing a curvaceous and sturdy-framed woman like myself.

You're not getting older... you're getting heavier

Marilyn Monroe aside, the sad truth is that as we age, body water, bone density, and muscle mass all tend to decrease, while body fat increases. We can fight this by keeping our hydration and bone density as high as possible, and by maintaining and building our muscle mass as we age. Sounds simple, doesn't it? If it were truly simple, more of us would be doing it, wouldn't we? Hopefully the tips below will make it as easy as possible.

Trade in fad diets for fitness

Most experts and chronic dieters can agree on one thing—dieting doesn't work. When tempted by new diets out there, remember this—quick weight loss tends to break down lean body tissue (muscles and organ tissue). Weight regain tends to put on body fat, which is exactly the opposite of what we want to happen. The more you lose weight and gain it back, the more difficult it's going to be to lose that weight again. If you've lost weight and gained it back several times...then you know exactly what I'm talking about.

If we changed our goal from losing weight to gaining health, we would be better off. To gain health we simply focus on eating healthy and getting regular exercise. To help us do this, it is essential we remember two things: You don't have to be thin to be fit and healthy, and a healthy weight is weight you are able to maintain without too much effort.

Get in a health mindset

If you focus on losing pounds, you immediately put yourself in a dieting mindset. You will likely fall into the weighing-yourself-daily failure trap. Change your focus to being and feeling healthy. I believe in eating and exercising for the health of it...and let the pounds fall where they may.

Don't give up just because you have the fat gene

We can't do anything about the genetic factors that influence obesity. On the other hand, we can't let our genes get in the way of our feeling good and being healthy. Your genes do enhance your susceptibility to gain weight in times of feast (versus famine), particularly when "feasting" with a high-fat diet. But if we eat a more healthful, moderate-fat diet, with lots of plant foods, and we get active and physically fit we are going to temper our genetic tendency to being overweight.

We can also work on some of the other factors that influence obesity—such as the behavioral and psychological factors that influence our particular lives. We can look at our eating habits, and what might be triggering us to overeat at times. If it looks like you have some issues with dieting, food, and body image, it might be a good idea to work with a psychologist or specially trained counselor to help you work through your particular past (so you can get on with your future). By the way, many people have long standing issues with food so please don't feel alone in this.

I know what it's like to have the fat gene on both sides of the family tree. My sisters and I have never been thin. But we were athletes through much of our youth and that helped us concentrate on what really mattered— health.

Take inventory of your eating habits

The one area you might need to look at more closely is changing the habits that might be leading you to excess weight. Do you have any unhealthy habits? Take the quiz below and find out:

The "What's Your Habit?" quiz

- Do you snack on sweets and chips more than fresh fruit and vegetables?
- Do you eat everything on your plate every time, thinking you would be wasting food if you didn't?
- Do you find yourself eating when you aren't really hungry because you are under stress, bored, angry, or upset? (Research indicates that using food to soothe feelings may be one big reason many people who lose weight gain it back.)
- Do you think you are being "bad" when you have your favorite foods? Do you think you must give them up in order to lose weight?
- Do you sometimes sit down for a small snack and end up eating a whole box of cookies, bag of chips, or small carton of ice cream?
- Do you sometimes let yourself get too hungry because you are trying to lose weight by not eating, even when you are hungry?
- Do you eat a lot of food late at night?

Now trade in these destructive habits for the following healthful habits:

1. Do you eat when you are hungry and stop when you are comfortable (not full)?
2. Do you eat mostly plant foods, making sure you get at least five servings of fruits and vegetables every day?

3. Do you drink alcohol only on occasion (or not at all)? When you do drink, do you keep it to no more than one drink a day?

4. If there is a certain food you really want, and you are physically hungry, do you have it in a small but satisfying portion?

5. Are you trying to eat more fiber-rich foods (fruits, vegetables, whole grains) and more balanced meals and snacks, including some protein and fat (mostly monounsaturated fat) because this generally makes meals more satisfying and staves off hunger longer?

6. Do you eat light at night, knowing you will be more comfortable sleeping if you aren't full, waking up hungry and ready to start your day?

7. Do you exercise regularly because you know it is important for your overall health?

8. Do you avoid distractions—such as reading or watching television—when you eat? Do you try to eat slowly and savor the taste of food?

9. Do you find other ways to comfort yourself when you are bored, stressed, angry or upset (such as going for a walk, calling a friend, listening to some uplifting music, or taking a bubble bath)? Don't ignore your feelings—find healthier ways of dealing with them. It's easier said than done, but get professional counseling with this if you need it.

10. Do you weigh yourself only when in doctors' offices because you know that the numbers on the scale really don't matter? What matters most is your overall health and how you feel.

Eat when you are hungry and stop when you are comfortable

This is a big key to nourishing yourself. Don't forget this. It's important. Everything about dieting goes against this. Dieting tells you, "don't listen to your hunger...follow our plan." Then it is more likely that you won't listen to your "I'm satisfied" or "I'm comfortable" cues and you might start overeating.

Know your food triggers

Many of us have developed certain triggers (environmental or emotional) that contribute to habits of overeating. Figuring out what your triggers are is a first, really important step towards squelching overeating. When your next food craving strikes, (especially if you aren't physically hungry at the time) try to figure out what brought it on. Use this chart to help you along.

Sensory Triggers:

Things you see, smell, taste that make you want to eat. (Television commercials, walking past a particular restaurant, etc.)

_____

_____

_____

Verbal Triggers:

Things you hear that make you want to eat. (Hearing someone talk about how great something tastes, someone telling you you've gained weight.)

_____

_____

_____

Emotional Triggers:

The psychological state or feelings that increase your desire to eat. (Being anxious, depressed, happy, or bored.)

_____

_____

_____

Other triggers:

Anything else that triggers cravings for certain foods when you aren't physically hungry.

_____

_____

_____

Maximize your calorie burning

Should you eat fewer calories? Yes, but that isn't very much fun. Your body needs more of a variety of nutrients as you age. If you eat less, you aren't likely to be getting more of these nutrients (calcium, vitamin D, antioxidants, vitamin B-12, zinc, and so on). There are many benefits to the suggestions below. You are truly better off burning more calories. Here's how:

1. **Exercising.** Exercising, in general, helps increase the number of calories you burn in a day. Of course we know we burn the extra calories while we exercise, but some new evidence suggests we even burn extra calories after we exercise (possibly for four to 12 hours after exercise). When you begin to exercise regularly, you use mostly glucose (carbohydrate) as your main fuel during aerobic exercise. Once you get into a regular exercise program and your body becomes fit, it will start to burn fat for the extra energy you need while you are exercising. Generally after exercising 20 minutes, the experienced exerciser is primarily burning fat for fuel. Go for at least 20 minutes of valuable fat-burning time, then you want to strive for those aerobic workouts that go for at least 40 minutes.

2. **Build muscle to burn more calories.** Muscle cells burn more calories at rest than fat cells do. How many calories are we talking about? About 70 percent of the calories you burn in a day are due to the metabolic activity of your lean body mass (muscle). If you want to build muscle tissue instead of fat tissue, exercise

has to be part of your plan. For best results use a combination of aerobic conditioning and strength training, especially during and after menopause.

3. **Eat breakfast.** Your metabolism (the rate at which the body burns calories) may slow down to conserve fuel. One of the biggest gaps in eating is when we sleep. If you are one of those people who isn't hungry right when you wake up, drink a small glass of juice or milk and then pack some food to bring with you wherever you go. When your hunger kicks in an hour or two later, you will be prepared.

4. **Eat small, frequent meals through the day and eat light at night.** Each time you eat, you set your body's digestive process in motion. Each time you start it up, you burn calories. The more frequently you eat, the more calories you burn just by digesting your food.

5. **Burn more calories digesting high-carbohydrate foods.** Your body uses more energy (burns more calories) to metabolize carbohydrates than it does to break down dietary fat. For example, if you eat 100 high-fat calories from potato chips over your calorie needs, about 97 of the 100 calories will probably end up as fat storage. But if you eat 100 higher carbohydrate calories from a baked potato, for example, 77 calories will probably be deposited as fat (because your body burned 23 calories to digest, convert, and store carbohydrate calories).

How to maintain your muscle mass

Muscle mass and muscle strength also decline as you age, because you start losing more and more muscle fibers and nerves that stimulate them. But you enhance your muscle mass through strength training and regular exercise. In terms of diet, you should make sure you are getting enough protein—but not too much. The only true way to build muscle is to use muscle.

Start strength training today!

Anyone can start boosting muscle mass by doing appropriate strength training exercises two or three times a week. You may have heard of these other terms for strength training: resistance training, weight training, and isotonics. Strength-training exercises usually involve activities that you repeat eight to 12 times in a row while standing or sitting in one place. The exercises pull a muscle (or set of muscles) to exhaustion. This encourages the muscle to grow and improve its tone. Strength training can be done two to three times a week for 30 to 40 minutes each session. Here are four great reasons to start strength training ASAP:

1. Strength training builds muscle mass. Because muscle mass requires more calories to sustain itself than body fat, strength training helps raise your metabolic rate.
2. Strength training increases bone density so it also helps reduce the risk of osteoporosis.
3. Strength training can ease the pain of osteoarthritis and may even ease the pain of rheumatoid arthritis.
4. The more muscle you have, the less insulin is required to get sugar from the blood to body tissues. Strength training helps reduce your risk of developing diabetes in your later years.

So why are Americans getting heavier?

The weight tables keep coming out. More diet books keep getting published. New drugs (herbal and otherwise) keep coming on the market. And we are only getting heavier. What's going on?

Does it come down to calories?

With all the new fat-free cookies and "light" products out there, how did this weight surplus happen? We are now in a culture where food is fast. Many of us eat out more than we eat in. Sweets are all around us. Soda is the number one source of added sugars.

As a nation we have become very aware of low fat diets and because of this we have been eating more fat free and low fat products. What we don't realize is that in many of these products, sugar is being substituted for the fat—with the calories staying pretty much the same. So we have really been trading fat for sugar. If we are of the mindset that we can eat more because it's fat-free, then we are actually eating more (and getting more calories) with some of the products.

Surveys have shown that we are getting a smaller percentage of our calories from fat than we were 15 to 20 years ago, but that we are eating more calories and more added sugars. We are actually eating 300 more calories a day when you compare data between 1975 and 1995. Not good—especially when you factor in that we are less active than we were back then.

Reducing dietary fat alone, without reducing calories, is not going to encourage weight loss. But as you reduce food fat along with reducing carbohydrates, calories will decrease and weight loss will be possible.

If we ate more fruits, vegetables, beans, and whole grains we would be eating fewer calories per a certain volume of food. This is compared to our higher meats and sweets type of diet.

If eating less fat is making us fatter, should we eat more fat to lose weight?

First of all, it is a myth. We aren't really eating less fat. Although Americans consume fewer "percent calories from fat" the actual number of grams that we take in has increased from 81 to 83 grams a day. This is because we have been eating more calories. So what's the difference between eating 81 and 83 grams of fat a day, you say?

This comes out to an extra:
- 18 extra fat calories a day.
- 126 extra fat calories a week.
- 540 extra fat calories a month.
- 6,500 extra fat calories a year.

 **Chapter 6**

Recipes You Cannot Live Without

W e know we should be eating more fruits, vegetables, whole grains, beans, and fish, but we can't seem to make it happen. I wanted to put together quick recipes that were packed with these nutrition powerhouses, but tasty enough that you actually look forward to eating them. Deep down your body knows what it needs. It will want to make many of these recipes again and again.

Granted, this chapter is not meant to be the answer to all your recipe woes. It is just a sampling to get you started. I have written two cookbooks that might also come in handy: *The Recipe Doctor* (a collection of recipes from my national column), and *Chez Moi* (lightening up recipes from famous restaurants).

Please note: The following is a key to the abbreviations used in the recipes: tablespoon [tbs.], teaspoon [tsp.], gram [g.], milligram [mg.], ounces [oz.], pound [lb.], and retinol equivalents (for vitamin A) [RE].

Recipes to inspire you to eat whole grains every day...

 ## Grilled Cheese on Wheat

This is one of the easiest ways to work a couple of whole grain servings into your day. Serve this as a quick weekday dinner with a nice cup of vegetable or bean soup and a bowl of fruit salad. Want to get a little fancy? Try the provolone pesto turkey sandwich suggestion below.

Makes 1 sandwich.

- 2 slices of whole wheat bread (make sure it is "whole" wheat).
- canola cooking spray.
- 1 oz. reduced fat cheese of choice (or use a 21 gram slice of Tilamook Cheddar or Kraft Deluxe American slices).

1. Start heating a thick non-stick frying pan over medium-low heat.
2. Spray the tops of two slices of whole wheat bread with canola cooking spray.
3. Lay one slice, sprayed side down, on the frying pan. Place slice of cheese on top, then place the second piece of bread (sprayed side up this time) on top of the cheese.
4. When bottom is nicely brown, flip sandwich over carefully to lightly brown the other side.

Per serving: 251 calories, 14.5 g. protein, 33 g. carbohydrate, 7.7 g. fat, 3.7 g. saturated fat, 15 mg. cholesterol, 5 g. fiber, 518 mg. sodium. Calories from fat: 27 percent.

Note 1: For a fancy rendition of a grilled cheese sandwich—a provolone pesto turkey grilled sandwich—use provolone cheese, spread one side of the bread with a teaspoon or two of pesto, and top with an ounce or two of thinly sliced turkey breast.

Note 2: Make an herbed grilled cheese sandwich just by spreading a little garlic-herb spread (such as Alouette Light) lightly on the inside of the top piece of bread before placing it in the pan.

 ## Quick Cereal Parfait

This is a fun, different way to work in your serving of whole grain cereal. I make this when I need a substantive snack in the late afternoon.

Makes 1 serving.

- 3/4 cup whole grain cereal of choice. (I like using raisin bran, Grape Nuts, or granola.)
- 1/2 cup yogurt, flavor of choice. (I like using lemon, berry, or vanilla.)
- 1/2 cup fruit of choice. (I like using berries.)

1. Spoon 1/4 cup of cereal into the bottom of a tall see-through glass. Then spoon 1/4 cup of the yogurt and 1/4 cup of fruit on top.
2. Repeat the layers with 1/4 cup of cereal, 1/4 cup of yogurt, and 1/4 cup of fruit. Finish with the remaining 1/4 cup of cereal.

Per serving (using Grape Nuts as the cereal): 260 calories, 9 g. protein, 54.5 g. carbohydrate, 3 g. fat, .8 g. saturated fat, 5 mg. cholesterol, 5.5 g. fiber, 212 mg. sodium. Calories from fat: 9 percent.

Vitamin A, 272 RE; vitamin C, 16 mg; folic acid, 127 mcg; calcium, 200 mg.

 ## Quick and Savory Brown Rice

This is one of those recipes I love to make again and again. It's quick and it complements chicken and fish entrees very well.

It uses brown rice (although you barely realize that you're eating brown rice—maybe that's why I like it so much).

Makes 6 side servings.

- 5 tsp. extra virgin olive oil.
- 1 cup long grain brown rice.
- 1/3 cup finely chopped green pepper.
- 1/3 cup finely chopped onion.
- 2 cups double strength (or condensed) chicken broth (beef or vegetable broth may also be used).
- 1 cup sliced mushrooms.
- 1/8 tsp. paprika.

1. Start heating olive oil over medium heat in a medium saucepan. Stir in rice and cook for 3 to 4 minutes or until lightly toasted (stir frequently to keep from burning).
2. Add green pepper and onion. Cook for about a minute and a half.
3. Stir in the chicken broth, mushrooms, and paprika. Bring to a boil, reduce heat to simmer, and cover pan.
4. After about 25 minutes, check whether the water has been absorbed and rice looks ready. Remove from stove and enjoy!

Per serving: 170 calories, 5 g. protein, 26 g. carbohydrate, 5.2 g. fat, .8 g. saturated fat, 0 mg. cholesterol, 1.5 g. fiber, 320 mg. sodium. Calories from fat: 28 percent.

Vitamin A, 4 RE; vitamin C, 6 mg.; folic acid, 14 mcg.; calcium, 13 mg.

 # Carrot Cake Bran Muffins

There are two types of recipes that I am most often asked to lighten up by people reading my column, The Recipe Doctor—bran muffins and carrot cake. I decided to put these two together and create a carrot cake bran muffin. I figured I couldn't go wrong this way!

Makes 12 (4 oz.) muffins.

- 1 cup crushed pineapple with juice (crushed pineapple canned in juice).
- 1/4 cup canola oil.
- 1 large egg, beaten lightly.
- 2 egg whites (1/4 cup liquid egg whites).
- 2 cups fat-free sour cream.
- 1/2 cup maple syrup. (Pancake syrup can be substituted.)
- 1 cup finely shredded or grated carrot.
- 2 cup unbleached flour.
- 2 tsp. baking powder.
- 2 tsp. baking soda.
- 1/2 tsp. salt.
- 2 cups 100 percent bran cereal.

1. Preheat oven to 400 degrees. Line pan with muffin papers. Coat inside of papers with a quick squirt of canola cooking spray.
2. In large bowl with electric mixer, cream together the pineapple with juice, canola oil, egg, egg whites, sour cream, and maple syrup until mixture is light and fluffy. Stir in grated carrots.
3. In a bowl, whisk together flour, baking powder, baking soda, salt, and bran cereal.
4. Beating on low speed, add bran mixture to sour cream mixture—just until combined (batter will be a little lumpy). Spoon batter by 1/2-cup increments into prepared muffin pan.
5. Bake in center of preheated oven for about 20 minutes or until they are golden brown and springy to the touch.

Per muffin: 248 calories, 7 g. protein, 44.5 g. carbohydrate, 5.7 g. fat, .5 g. saturated fat, 18 mg. cholesterol, 4.5 g. fiber, 505 mg. sodium. Calories from fat: 20 percent.

Vitamin A, 324 RE; vitamin C, 13 mg.; folic acid, 17 mcg.; calcium, 120 mg.

Recipes to inspire you to eat more cabbage family vegetables...

 ## Quick Vegetable Bean Salad

One serving of this quick salad gives you a dose of alpha and beta carotene, folic acid, vitamin C, fiber (and plant omega-3 fatty acids from the canola oil). If you want to make this more of a meal and you want to add fish omega-3 fatty acids and some protein into the picture, stir in a can of albacore tuna.

Makes 8 servings.

- 3 cups baby carrots, or diced or thinly sliced carrots.
- 3 cups broccoli florets cut into bite-sized pieces.
- 15 oz. can kidney beans, rinsed and drained well.
- 1/2 cup finely chopped mild onion (use less if desired).
- 1/2 cup 1/3-less-fat bottled vinaigrette made with canola or olive oil. (I use Seven Seas 1/3-less-fat Red Wine Vinaigrette with canola).
- 6 oz. can albacore tuna canned in water (optional).

1. Add carrot pieces to microwave-safe covered dish with 1/4 cup water and cook on HIGH about 3 to 5 minutes (or until just barely tender). Drain well and add to medium-sized serving bowl.
2. Add broccoli pieces to microwave-safe covered dish with 1/4 cup water and cook on HIGH about 3 to 5 minutes (or until just barely tender). Drain well and add to medium-sized serving bowl.
3. Add beans, chopped onion, and vinaigrette (and tuna if desired) to serving bowl and toss well to blend.

Per serving: 110 calories, 5 g. protein, 19 g. carbohydrate, 2.5 g. fat, 0 g. saturated fat, 0 mg. cholesterol, 7 g. fiber, 310 mg. sodium. Calories from fat: 20 percent.
Vitamin A, 1,568 RE; folic acid, 70 mcg.; vitamin C, 51 mg.

Extra-Creamy Coleslaw

Some people only eat cabbage when they eat coleslaw. For them, here's a reduced fat version from a favorite fast food chicken chain.

Makes 8 servings.

- 3 tbs. sugar.
- 1/2 tsp. salt.
- 1/8 tsp. freshly ground pepper.
- 1/4 cup 1 percent milk.
- 2 tbs. Best Foods mayonnaise (or similar).
- 1/3 cup fat-free (or "light") sour cream.
- 1/4 cup low-fat buttermilk.
- 1 1/2 tbs. white vinegar or rice vinegar.
- 2 tbs. lemon juice.
- 8 cups finely chopped cabbage (about 1 medium head).
- 1 cup grated carrots.

1. In a large bowl, blend the sugar, salt, pepper, milk, mayonnaise, sour cream, buttermilk, vinegar, and lemon juice with an electric mixer until smooth. Spoon it into a large bowl.
2. Add in the carrots and cabbage. Toss to blend with dressing.
3. Cover and refrigerate for at least 3 hours before serving.

Per serving: 81 calories, 2 g. protein, 12.5 g. carbohydrate, 3 g. fat, .5 g. saturated fat, 2 mg. cholesterol, 2 g. fiber, 182 mg. sodium. Calories from fat: 32 percent.
Vitamin A, 418 RE; vitamin C, 25 mg.; folic acid, 33 mcg.; calcium, 60 mg.

 ## Cauliflower Au Gratin

I'm not too keen on cauliflower myself, but I could eat a whole bowl of this stuff. Granted it has more calories and grams of fat than a bowl of steamed cauliflower, but this is the type of recipe that will make a cauliflower fan out of just about anyone who tries it.

Makes 3 large servings (6 small).

- 1 head cauliflower (about 6 cups raw cauliflower bite-sized florets).
- 2 tbs. chopped shallots.
- 1 tbs. minced garlic.
- 1 cup vegetable or chicken broth.
- 1 cup whole milk. (Land O'Lakes fat-free half-and-half can also be used.)
- 1 tsp. horseradish (add more to taste).
- salt and freshly ground pepper to taste.
- 1/2 cup packed grated "light" Jarlsberg or "light" Swiss cheese. (Gruyere can also be used.)

1. Preheat oven to 350 degrees. Coat a 9" pie plate with canola cooking spray.
2. Cut cauliflower into small florets (coarsely chop the stems and hold on to them for later), and blanch the florets in boiling, salted water until tender (about 2 minutes). Remove from heat and drain.
3. Start to heat a thick, nonstick frying pan or skillet to medium-low and coat the pan with canola cooking spray. Add the coarsely chopped cauliflower stems, shallots, and garlic, and gently sauté until soft (do not brown). Add the broth and cook until the stock is almost gone.
4. Pour this mixture, with the milk and horseradish, into a food processor or blender. Pulse until fairly smooth. Season with salt and pepper to taste.
5. Spread the cauliflower florets into the prepared pie plate and pour the milk mixture over the top. Gently toss to blend.
6. Sprinkle the cheese over the top. Bake until golden brown (about 15 to 18 minutes).

Per large serving: 170 calories, 13 g. protein, 18 g. carbohydrate, 6.5 g. fat, 3.5 g. saturated fat, 20 mg. cholesterol, 4 g.

fiber, 530 mg. sodium. Calories from fat: 22 percent.
Vitamin A, 65 RE; vitamin C, 95 mg.; folic acid, 123 mcg.; calcium, 288 mg.

Recipes to inspire you to eat more beans...

 ## Black Bean Nacho Dip

This is wonderful served with fresh flour tortillas or reduced fat tortilla chips.

Makes 4 servings.

- 1/2 cup chopped onion.
- 2 garlic cloves, chopped.
- 1 tbs. olive oil.
- 2 tsp. chili powder.
- 15 oz. can black beans, rinsed and drained.
- 1/8 cup beef broth. (Non-alcoholic beer or water can also be used.)
- 1/2 tsp. cumin seeds.
- Cayenne red pepper to taste.
- 4 oz. reduced-fat Jack cheese, grated.
- Salt to taste.

Garnish:

- 1 ripe tomato, chopped.
- 1 tbs. chopped fresh cilantro.
- 1 tbs. finely chopped jalapeno pepper (optional).
- 1/2 cup fat-free or "light" sour cream.

1. Preheat oven to 450 degrees. Lightly coat a small, shallow baking dish with canola cooking spray (a 9" loaf pan will also work).
2. In a medium saucepan, sauté the onion and garlic in the oil until clear. Sprinkle with chili powder and cook 1 minute longer. Add the beans and broth and cook

until the mixture thickens (about 4 minutes).

3. Mash the beans with potato masher until the mixture is half smooth and half chunky. Add the cumin seeds. Season to taste with salt and cayenne. Spoon mixture into prepared dish, top with grated cheese, and bake or microwave until the cheese melts. Remove from oven. Spread sour cream over the top and sprinkle top with tomatoes, cilantro and diced jalapeno if desired.

Per serving: 228 calories, 16 g. protein, 24 g. carbohydrate, 8 g. fat, 3 g. saturated fat, 15 mg. cholesterol, 6.5 g. fiber, 400 mg. sodium. Calories from fat: 30 percent.
Vitamin A, 117 RE; vitamin C, 8 mg.; folic acid, 12 mcg.; calcium, 284 mg.

 ## Savory Slow Cooker Chili

Chili is one of the most popular ways to eat beans, so I wanted to make sure you had a good and quick recipe for one. One of the easiest ways to make chili is to brown the meat and onions and throw everything in a slow cooker to simmer, unattended, all day. The original recipe calls for ground chuck, but you could use a ground sirloin (or super lean ground beef), leftover chicken breast cut into bite-sized pieces, or even chunks of sautéed or smoked tofu.

Makes 6 servings.

*   1 lb. diet, super lean ground beef or ground sirloin (2 cups of skinless, roasted chicken, cut into bite-sized pieces works great too).
*   1 tbs. canola oil.
*   1 large onion, chopped.
*   2 cloves garlic, crushed or minced.
*   Salt to taste.
*   1/4 tsp. cayenne red pepper.
*   1/4 tsp. dried oregano.
*   1/4 tsp. ground cumin.

- 1 to 2 tbs. chili powder, depending on "heat" preference.
- 2 (14-oz.) cans stewed tomatoes, undrained.
- 14 oz. can tomato sauce.
- 2 (16-oz.) cans red kidney beans, rinsed and drained.

1. If using ground beef, add the meat to large skillet and brown, breaking up lumps and cooking until brown. Add onion and garlic and cook until onion is limp (add canola oil if needed to prevent mixture from sticking to pan).

   If using roasted chicken, add canola oil to large skillet and add onion and garlic and cook over medium-low heat until onion is limp. Stir in roasted chicken pieces and cook another minute or two.

2. Add browned beef or chicken mixture to slow cooker along with cayenne red pepper, oregano, cumin, chili powder. Stewed tomatoes, tomato sauce, and beans. Stir, cover, and set slow cooker to LOW (and let simmer 8 hours) or on HIGH (and let simmer 3 to 4 hours). Taste for seasoning and correct if necessary.

3. Spoon into serving bowls and sprinkle each serving with grated reduced-fat cheddar or Jack cheese if desired.

Per serving (with chicken): 274 calories, 24 g. protein, 35 g. carbohydrate, 4.5 g. fat, .7 g. saturated fat, 40 mg. cholesterol, 12 g. fiber, 508 mg. sodium. Calories from fat: 15 percent.
Vitamin A, 93 RE; vitamin C, 21 mg.; folic acid, 92 mcg.; calcium, 87 mg.

Per serving (with super lean ground beef): 292 calories, 21 g. protein, 35 g. carbohydrate, 8 g. fat, 2.3 g. saturated fat, 26 mg. cholesterol, 12 g. fiber, 514 mg. sodium. Calories from fat: 25 percent.
Vitamin A, 90 RE; vitamin C, 21 mg.; folic acid, 95 mcg.; calcium, 84 mg.

Rosemary Bean Salad

This simple but tasty dish is named after the herb, which adds a wonderful flavor. It uses canned beans so it takes only minutes to make.

Makes 5 (1/3 cup) servings.

- 16-oz. can white beans (or navy beans), rinsed and drained.
- 2 oz. jar chopped pimientos, drained.
- 2 cloves garlic, minced.
- 1/2 tsp. ground black pepper.
- 1 tbs. olive oil.
- 2 tbs. red wine or sherry vinegar.
- 2 tbs. capers.
- 1 1/2 tsp. chopped fresh rosemary (or 1/2 tsp. dried).
- Romaine lettuce leaves.
1. Combine the white beans, pimiento, garlic, pepper, olive oil, vinegar, capers, and rosemary in a bowl; mix well.
2. Spoon each serving of bean salad onto a romaine lettuce leaf on each dinner or lunch plate.

Per serving: 116 calories, 6 g. protein, 18.3 g. carbohydrate, 2.5 g. fat, .4 g. saturated fat, 0 mg. cholesterol, 4.4 g. fiber, 107 mg. sodium. Calories from fat: 19 percent.

Vitamin A, 79 RE; Vitamin C, 13 mg.; folic acid, 77 mcg.; calcium, 68 mg.

Recipes that use antioxidant- and/or folic-acid-rich fruits or vegetables

 Apricot-Orange Smoothie

This great tasting drink pumps up your morning with some calcium and carotene phytochemicals too! Stir in some flaxseed for a boost of soluble fiber, omega-3 fatty acids, and phytoestrogens.

Makes 2 servings.

- 15 oz. can of chunky apricots in light syrup. (I use S&W Almond Recipe Sun Apricots.)
- 6 oz. vanilla yogurt (custard style works great).
- 1 cup orange juice. (Calcium-fortified orange juice is now available in cartons).
- 2 cups ice cubes.
- 1-2 tbs. ground flaxseed (if desired).

1. Add all the ingredients to a blender.
2. Blend for about 5 to 8 seconds until smooth.

Per serving: 250 calories, 6 g. protein, 57 g. carbohydrate, 1.5 g. fat, .7 g. saturated fat, 4 mg. cholesterol, 2.5 g. fiber, 65 mg. sodium. Calories from fat: 5 percent.

Vitamin A, 300 RE; folic acid, 50 mcg.; vitamin C, 68mg.

 Tropical Island Smoothie

Makes 2 smoothies.

- 1 cup papaya or mango chunks (frozen, bottled, or fresh).
- 1 cup pineapple juice. If you don't care for pineapple, substitute another juice.
- 1 banana, sliced.
- 6 oz. container lime yogurt. (Pineapple or other flavor can be used.)
- 2 cups ice cubes.

1. Add all the ingredients to a blender.
2. Blend for about 5 to 8 seconds until smooth.

Per serving: 230 calories, 4 g. protein, 51 g. carbohydrate, 2 g. fat, .5 g. saturated fat, 5 mg. cholesterol, 2.5 g. fiber, 44 mg. sodium. Calories from fat: 8 percent.

Vitamin A, 25 RE; vitamin C, 62 mg.; folic acid, 66 mcg.; calcium, 200 mg.

Fancy Fruit Salad

This tastes as beautiful as it looks. You can use a combination of fresh and canned fruits so it is easier to make and more of a year-round recipe.

Makes 6 servings.
- 8 cups of assorted fruit pieces, for example:
- 2 cups melon balls or chunks (such as cantaloupe).
- 1 1/4 cups sliced peaches. (15-oz. can of light peaches, drained, can be substituted.)
- 1 1/4 cups cut-up pears. (15-oz. can of light pears, drained and cut, can be substituted.)
- 1 cup raspberries, rinsed and drained.
- 1 1/2 cups bite-size pieces of apple.
- 1 cup seedless grapes.
- 1-2 tbs. sugar.
- 1-2 tbs. liqueur of choice: Grand Marnier, Caravella, amaretto, etc.

1. Combine the various fruit in a serving bowl. Sprinkle the sugar and liqueur over the top and gently toss to blend well.
2. Cover and refrigerate at least 2 hours. Mix again before serving.

Per serving: 114 calories, 1 g. protein, 28 g. carbohydrate, .5 g. fat, 0 g. saturated fat, 0 mg. cholesterol, 3.5 g. fiber, 5 mg. sodium. Calories from fat: 5 percent.
Vitamin A, 150 RE, vitamin C, 30 mg., folic acid, 17 mcg., calcium, 20 mg.

You'll fall in love with the look of dark green spinach, matched with bright red strawberries and wonderful raspberry poppy seed dressing drizzled all over it. You can substitute romaine lettuce for the spinach if you prefer—they both are rich sources of folic acid (romaine contains 76 mcg. of folic acid per cup; spinach contains 58 mcg. per cup).

Strawberry Spinach Salad

AU: How many servings?
- 8 cups fresh spinach or romaine lettuce, thoroughly washed, dried and torn, lightly packed.
- 3 cups fresh strawberries, cleaned, hulled, and halved (2 to 3 cups).

Quick Dressing:
- 2 tbs. canola oil.
- 2 tbs. rice vinegar or cider vinegar.
- 2 tbs. honey or light corn syrup.
- 1 tbs. sesame seeds.
- 1 1/2 tsp. poppy seeds.
- 1 tsp. minced onion.
- 1/8 tsp. Worcestershire sauce.
- 1/8 tsp. paprika.

1. Add spinach and strawberries to large serving bowl. (Do not mix.)
2. Add dressing ingredients to a blender or food processor and blend until thoroughly mixed and thickened. (Do not over mix.)
3. Just before serving, toss the salad gently with only the amount of dressing it takes to coat the spinach and strawberries nicely.

Per serving: 104 calories, 3 g. protein, 13 g. carbohydrate, 5.5 g. fat, .4 g. saturated fat, 0 mg. cholesterol, 63 mg. sodium. Calories from fat: 45 percent.

Vitamin A, 503 RE; vitamin C, 52 mg.; folic acid, 157 mcg.; calcium, 97 mg.

Antipasto Veggies

This is a fun, quick way to zest up your veggies. Blend the vinaigrette in a self-sealing plastic bag, add the veggies, shake, and leave overnight or several hours in the refrigerator.

Makes 8 servings.

(**Note:** To skip a step, substitute 2/3 cup of reduced-fat bottled vinaigrette that uses olive oil or canola oil and contains around 5 grams of fat per 2-tablespoon serving [there are several on the market].)

Vinaigrette:
- 1/3 cup seasoned rice vinegar or other vinegar.
- 1/3 cup apple juice.
- 2 tbs. olive oil.
- 2 tbs. lemon juice.
- 2 tsp. Dijon mustard.
- 1/4 cup finely chopped green onion.
- 2 tbs. snipped parsley or 2 tsp. dried parsley flakes.
- 2 cloves garlic, minced.
- 1 tsp. dried thyme flakes.
- salt and pepper to taste.

Veggies:
- 3 cups broccoli florets, steamed or cooked in the microwave until just barely tender. (Do not overcook.)
- 2 cups asparagus spears, steamed or cooked in the microwave until just barely tender.
- 2 cups cauliflower florets, steamed or cooked in the microwave until just barely tender.
- 3 tomatoes, cut into quarters, or about 15 cherry tomatoes.

1. Lightly cook all the veggies if you haven't already done so (except the tomatoes).
2. Add the bottled vinaigrette (or vinaigrette ingredients) to a gallon size self-sealing bag. Seal and shake gently to

blend the vinaigrette ingredients. Add salt and pepper to taste. Shake to blend.

3. Add the veggies (except tomatoes) to the bag and close the bag. Shake gently to cover the veggies with the dressing. Refrigerate in bag several hours or overnight, turning occasionally.

4. Remove the vegetables with a slotted spoon and arrange on a serving platter. Add the tomatoes to the bag and gently toss to coat tomatoes with vinaigrette. Remove with slotted spoon, and arrange on serving platter with the other veggies.

Per serving: (including half the vinaigrette) 59 calories, 3.5 g. protein, 9 g. carbohydrate, 2.2 g. fat, .3 g. saturated fat, 0 mg. cholesterol, 3.5 g. fiber, 25 mg. sodium. Calories from fat: 29 percent.

Vitamin A, 134 RE, vitamin C, 74 mg., folic acid, 99 mcg., calcium, 43 mg.

Recipes that inspire you to eat more fish...

 ## Honey Glazed Salmon

I love this recipe! It gives you melt-in-your-mouth salmon in minutes. It even works great in a toaster oven (which comes in handy in summer when you want to avoid overheating your kitchen).

Makes 2 servings.

- 12-14 oz. salmon fillet (tail end if possible because it has almost no bones).
- 3 tbs. honey.
- 1 tsp. olive oil.
- 2 tsp. lemon juice.

- 1/2 tsp. Italian seasoning (herb blend).
- 1/4 tsp. garlic powder or 1 minced or crushed garlic clove.
- A pinch or two black pepper.

1. Line 9" x 9" baking dish with foil and coat foil with canola cooking spray. If you are using a toaster oven, line the toaster oven pan with foil, then coat the foil with canola cooking spray.
2. Lay salmon fillet on the foil, skin side up, and broil (about 4 inches from the heat) for about 6 minutes.
3. Flip fish over and spread honey glazes evenly over salmon. Broil until salmon is cooked throughout (another 6 or so minutes).
4. Cut fillet into 2 servings and remove each serving from the pan (usually the skin can easily be separated from the fish at this point) and place on dinner plate.

Per serving: 272 calories, 27 g. protein, 18 g. carbohydrate, 10 g. fat, 1.5 g. saturated fat, 75 mg. cholesterol, 0 g. fiber, 60 mg. sodium. Calories from fat: 34 percent.

 ## Bourbon Basted Salmon

This marinade would be great for most types of fish. We thoroughly enjoyed it with salmon though. If you mix the marinade and add it to the fish in the morning, it will be ready to grill or broil when you come home from work.

Makes 4 servings.

- 1 1/2 lbs. salmon fillets (get the tail end if you can for fewer bones).
- 1/4 cup packed brown sugar.
- 3 tbs. bourbon whiskey (Scotch will work too).
- 3 tbs. light soy sauce (reduced sodium).
- 1 tbs. canola oil.

1. Place the salmon in a gallon size self-sealing plastic bag (or place the salmon skin side down in a shallow baking dish).

2. In a small bowl, combine all the other ingredients. Pour over the salmon in the bag (or dish) and marinate in the refrigerator for at least 1 hour.
3. Lift salmon out of the bag (reserve marinade). If using a grill or barbecue, cook fish directly on a grill that has been coated with canola cooking spray (over hot coals). Turn once, about 7 minutes per side. Baste with the reserve marinade if desired.

Note: To cook the salmon without a grill or barbecue, line a shallow baking dish (a 9" x 9" pan should do) with foil and spray foil with canola cooking spray. Set salmon on foil and brush some of the marinade over the top. Broil 6 inches from heat for about 7 minutes. Turn fillet over, baste with marinade and broil another 7 minutes or so or until fish is cooked throughout.

Per serving: 341 calories, 35 g. protein, 10.5 g. carbohydrate, 14 g. fat, 2 g. saturated fat, 93 mg. cholesterol, 0 g. fiber, 450 mg. sodium. Calories from fat: 38 percent.

 ## Champagne Snapper

Any recipe with the word "champagne" in it gets my attention. I happen to be a fan of the bubbly.

Makes 4 servings.
- 1 cup champagne or dry white wine (non-alcoholic can also be used).
- 1 tbs. butter.
- 1 bay leaf.
- 1/4 cup finely chopped fresh parsley.
- 2 tbs. finely chopped onion.
- 2 tbs. finely chopped celery.
- 2 tbs. fat-free half-and-half. (Whole milk can also be used.)
- 2 tsp. Wondra quick-mixing flour.
- 4 snapper fillets (sole or cod can be substituted).
- 1/2 tsp. salt (or to your preference).

- 1/2 tsp. freshly ground pepper (or to your preference).
- 1/2 cup sliced mushrooms.
- 2 tbs. freshly grated Parmesan cheese.

1. Preheat oven to 350 degrees. Coat a 13" x 9" baking dish with canola cooking spray.
2. Combine the champagne, butter, bay leaf, parsley, onion, and celery in a saucepan. Bring to a boil, reduce heat, and simmer until reduced by half. Remove the bay leaf. In a custard cup, blend the the cream or whole milk with the Wondra flour then stir into champagne mixture. Take the pan off the stove.
3. Dry the fish with paper toweling and sprinkle with salt and pepper. Arrange in one layer in the baking dish. Add the mushrooms to the sauce and pour the sauce evenly over the fillets. Sprinkle with cheese. Bake uncovered for 25 to 30 minutes, or until the top is browned.

Per serving: 235 calories, 31.5 g. protein, 2.5 g. carbohydrate, 5.8 g. fat, 2.8 g. saturated fat, 63 mg. cholesterol, .3 g. fiber, 425 mg. sodium. Calories from fat: 22 percent.

Vitamin A, 72 RE; vitamin C, 3 mg.; folic acid, 11 mcg.; calcium, 96 mg.

Deli-Style Albacore Tuna Sandwich

Makes 2 sandwiches.
- 6 1/2-oz. can albacore tuna (canned in spring water), drained.
- 2 tsp. mayonnaise (or canola mayonnaise).
- 2 tbs. fat-free sour cream (or "light" sour cream).
- 1/2 tsp. dill weed.
- 1/8 cup finely chopped celery.
- 1 tbs. sliced black olives (optional).
- salt and pepper to taste (salt is optional).

- 1/4 cup thinly sliced cucumber.
- 2 whole grain bagels or 4 slices whole grain bread.

1. Add tuna to small or medium bowl.
2. Add the mayonnaise, sour cream, dill, celery, and black olives if desired. Mix well and taste. Add salt and pepper to taste if desired.
3. Place half the mixture on a slice of wheat bread (or on half of a bagel). Lay sliced cucumbers over the top. Place other piece of bagel or bread on top.
4. Repeat with remaining tuna mixture, cucumbers, and bagel/bread.

Per serving: 297 calories, 29 g. protein, 35 g. carbohydrate, 5 g. fat, .9 g. saturated fat, 28 mg. cholesterol, 6 g. fiber, 600 mg. sodium. Calories from fat: 15 percent.

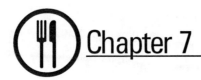 Chapter 7

Navigating the Supermarket

G enerally, the more you know about a food product, the better off you'll be. I know it sounds like you are going to be reading labels for hours every time you set foot in the supermarket. But keep in mind that most of us buy the same products over and over. What we really need is to invest some time initially. Once we have checked labels and surveyed some of our favorite products, we won't have to check those labels out again.

Start by reading the portion size on the label, because what the manufacturer considers a serving and what you think is a serving can be two very different things. I am continually amazed at some of the portion sizes I've found listed. A popular muffin company listed half a muffin as a serving (have you ever seen someone eat half of a muffin?). If I hadn't read the portion size on the label and just took a quick glance at the fat, fiber, sugar and calories, I would have thought the muffin had 12 grams of fat instead of 24 and 310 calories instead of 620! Some products within the same category even have different serving sizes. Some breads list one slice as a serving. Others use two slices. In the cereal aisle you'll find everything from half a cup to one and a half cups as a serving.

Once you've made it past the portion size, you can follow the label down to find calories, fat grams, saturated fat grams, fiber grams, and sugar grams.

Fat-free but full of calories

Just because a product is fat-free doesn't mean it is calorie-free or that you can eat the whole box in one sitting. In fact, many of these fat-free products have just as many calories as the full-fat versions. How can that be? In a word—sugar.

Sugar, whether it comes from honey, corn syrup, brown sugar, or high fructose corn syrup, can add moisture and help tenderize bakery products. When added to foods it adds flavor and structure. I'm not surprised that manufacturers have turned to sugar for assistance in developing reduced-fat and fat-free products. Keep in mind that although a majority of the fat-free and lower-fat products on the supermarket shelves have skimmed off the fat, the calories are mostly the same as the full-fat versions (saving only 10 or 20 calories per serving).

Some products have gone too far

I've got to confess a few of my product biases. I am philosophically opposed to fat-free margarine, mayonnaise, and cheese. If you take the fat completely out of a food that was mostly fat to begin with—such as mayonnaise, or butter—then what have you really got? Something other than mayonnaise and butter.

More than half of the new fat-free or "light" products I try end up in the garbage can. But about 20 percent of the products end up being keepers. These are the products that successfully found an optimal reduced level of fat. These are the foods that withstood a modest reduction in fat without a huge loss in taste satisfaction. You'll find them listed in this chapter.

Can't get any satisfaction?

I don't know if you've noticed this or not, but some of these fat-free products (many of which are really high in sugar) aren't very satisfying or filling in the long run. So if you are eating these foods, there is the tendency to eat more. This will only make you hungry again. When the low-fat, no-fat diets became the craze, products with more sugar and less fat proliferated. Now we have to rethink these choices. Ask yourself a few questions:

- Does this product have a lot of sugar? (Most of them do.)
- Does this fat-free product have almost as many calories as the regular version? (Most of them do.)
- Do I truly enjoy this product? Do I tend to eat unreasonable amounts of it to satisfy myself? (Most of you do.)

With the 10 food steps to freedom in mind, I've taken the liberty of reading some labels and putting together tables that I hope will save you from hours of label reading.

Whole grain products you'll want to know about

Basically, when it comes to whole grains in the supermarket, you'll need to go no further than the cereal and bread aisle. Oh sure, there's brown rice, barley, and such, but let's face it—most of us are going to be more likely to eat a whole grain bread or cereal product on an almost daily basis.

A whole grain has the bran and germ part of the grain intact. Each whole grain has its own set of phytochemicals though, and variety is the spice of life, so if you can find it in your recipe repertoire to work in some barley and brown rice occasionally—terrific! There's a fast and tasty recipe with brown rice in the recipe chapter to get you started.

- Barley was one of the first grains to be cultivated by man and is popular in Europe.
- Brown rice has the nutrient-dense bran portion of rice that is normally taken off to make white rice. I personally have been really happy with my recent attempts to substitute brown long grain rice for white.
- Buckwheat is the major whole grain in Japan used to make soba noodles.
- Millet is rarely used today but was once popular in Europe.
- Oats are one of the highest protein grains and one of the highest in soluble fiber too.
- Rye is a whole grain prized by German, Russian, and Scandinavian bread makers. Here we have two types of rye bread to choose from in our supermarkets and bakeries (dark and golden). Germany has more than one hundred different types of rye bread.

Whole grain breads and bagels

Buyer beware. Many of the breads that sound like they should have tons of fiber don't. You'd think something called "multigrain" should be able to provide a couple of measly grams of fiber per slice. Even trickier, there are a few breads that list the nutrition info per two slices, and the rest use one slice.

Some of the whole grain breads I found are on page 126.

Whole grain cereals

What really distinguishes one cereal from the next is not its fat and sodium content, but its grams of sugar and fiber. The cereals that have a lot more sugar are usually the ones that have a lot less fiber too. The table on page 127 lists the whole grain cereals with the most fiber.

Whole grain frozen waffles

There are three whole grain, frozen waffles on the market. Frozen waffles might not be your breakfast of choice, but topped

Whole grain breads and bagels

	Fiber (g)	Calories	Fat (g)
Breads (per 2 slices)			
EarthGrains:			
Country Hearth			
100% Whole Wheat	6	220	3
Mrs. Wright's:			
100% Whole Wheat	4	140	2
Northwest Grain Country:			
100% Whole Wheat	6	200	3
Early American	4	220	2
Oroweat:			
Light 100% whole wheat	7	80	0.5
Light Country Oat Bread	5	80	1
Light 9-Grain	5	80	0.5
100% Whole Wheat	4	180	2
Health Nut	4	200	4
Branola	4	180	2
Best winter wheat	4	180	6
Roman Meal:			
Sun grain bread	4	200	4
Dakota wheat bread	4	180	2
Bagel (per bagel)			
Oroweat:			
100% Whole Wheat	9	240	1.5
Oat Nut	4	270	4
Multi Grain	4	260	1.5

with some fresh fruit and a little berry syrup, and they're not a bad choice on a busy weekday morning.

Shopping for less sugar

In this country, we don't just have a sweet tooth—we have a sweet mouth! According to a recent USDA food consumption sur-

Best breakfast cereals

Type of cereal	Fiber (g)	Cal.	Sugar (g)	Fat (g)	Folic Acid (%DV)
Fiber One bran cereal, 1/2 cup	14	60	0	1	25%
All-Bran (100% bran cereal) thin strips, 1 cup	20	160	12	2	50%
Wheat Bran flakes, (Post) 1 1/2 cups	10	200	12	1	50%
Muesli[1] cereal (Safeway Select Healthy Advantage), 2/3 cup	8	190	15	3	25%
Raisin Bran flakes, 1 cup (Kellogg's)	8	190	18	1.5	25%
Multi-Grain Chex (with wheat, rice, and corn bran), 1 cup	7	200	12	1.5	25%
Shredded Wheat bite size Lightly sweetened[1] (Kellogg's), 1 cup	6	200	12	1	25%
Grape Nuts Whole Grain & Barley Flakes, 1 1/2 cups	6	220	10	2	50%
Grape Nuts Wheat & Barley crunchy Nuggets, 1/2 cup	5	210	7	1	25%
Wheat Chex (100% whole grain), 1 cup	5	180	5	1	25%
Toasted Oatmeal Squares (Quaker), 1 cup	4	210	9	2.5	100%
Lowfat granola, (Safeway Select Healthy Advantage), 2/3 cup	4	220	16	2.5	25%
Hot cereal:					
Wheatena (hot toasted wheat cereal), 1 cup	6.5	136	0	1	9%
Oatmeal, cooked, 1 cup	4	145	0	2	5%
Instant oatmeal maple flavor 1 packet (43 g)	3	160	13	2	20%

[1]Includes barley, whole wheat, wheat bran, oats, dates, raisins, and nuts.
[2]The unsweetened variety contains 170 calories, and 0 grams sugar.

Frozen Waffles

Waffles (2 per serving)	Fiber (g)	Cal.	Fat (g)
Eggo Nutri-Grain Multigrain	5	160	5
Eggo Nutri-Grain Whole Wheat	3	170	5
Eggo Golden Oat	3	140	2.5

vey, the average adult is eating about 20 teaspoons of added sugar every day. That computes to about 320 calories. If we would just cut this amount (from 20 teaspoons of added sugar a day to eight teaspoons) we could potentially trim 3500 calories a month, which translates to about 1.5 lost pounds per month.

If there is a dessert you really want, please enjoy it. People can refrain from overeating favorite foods if they give themselves the special foods they want from time to time. For all the days in between, here are some simple ways to cut some extra calories in the dessert department. Dessert can also be a great way to enjoy fruits. You'll notice many of the suggestions below give you ideas on how to include fruits.

Top 10 big ticket sugar sources

The latest data from the USDA's Continuing Survey of Food Intakes by individuals shows that the top food categories that contribute added sugar in women's diets are:

1. Carbonated soft drinks: 22.9%
2. Sugar and sugar substitute blends (table sugars): 6.8%
3. Fruit drinks: 6.1%
4. Cakes: 4.4%
5. Cookies: 4.3%
6. Candy (included chocolate): 4.%
7. Frozen milk desserts (includes ice cream and frozen yogurt): 3.7%
8. Tea (includes bottled teas): 3.7%
9. Syrup, honey, molasses, and other sweet toppings: 3.%
10. Yogurt: 2.4%

Sweet tooth selections

Choose...	Instead Of...
Starbucks Frappuccino (mocha) frozen coffee bar (1 bar=120 cal., 2 g. fat)	1/2 cup Starbucks Coffee Almond Fudge ice cream (250 cal., 13 g. fat)
Ben & Jerry's Chocolate Fudge Brownie low-fat frozen yogurt (1/2 cup=190 cal., 2.5 g. fat)	Fudge brownie a la mode (350 cal., 20 g. fat)
Reduced-Fat Chips Ahoy (3 cookies=140 cal., 5 g. fat)	Chunky Chips Ahoy (3 cookies=240 cal., 12 g. fat)
Snackwells Mint Crème cookies (2 cookies=110 cal., 3.5 g. fat)	Mystic Mint cookie or mint ice cream (2 cookies=180 cal., 9 g. fat)
3 Reduced Fat Oreo cookies with a glass of 1 percent low-fat milk (230 cal., 6 g. fat)	Cookies & Cream ice cream (1 cup) or a cookies & cream candy bar (ice cream=350 cal., 24 g. fat)
Jell-O instant chocolate pudding (Made with 2 percent milk) (1 serving=160 cal., 2.7 g fat)	Chocolate cream pie (1 small slice=305 cal., 16 g. fat)
Betty Crocker Low-Fat fudge brownie mix (1/18 pan=130 cal., 2.5 g. fat)	Regular fudge brownie (1/18 pan=175 cal., 9 g. fat)
Strawberries or other berries with 1/2 cup light vanilla ice cream (145 cal., 3.3 g. fat, 1.3 g. fiber)	1/2 cup ice cream (about 250 cal., 13 g. fat)
Lemon or coconut meringue pie (1/8 pie=240 cal., 8 g. fat)	Lemon or coconut cream pie (1/8 pie=415 cal., 22 g. fat)
Mrs. Smith's blackberry cobbler (1/8 cobbler=250 cal., 9 g. fat)	Mrs. Smith's berry pie (1/12 pie=330 cal., 15 g. fat)
1 piece angel food cake with 1/2 cup berries or other fruit (175 cal., 1 g. fat, plus 4 g. fiber)	1 thin piece frosted cake (275 cal., 12 g. fat)
Weight Watchers Smart Ones New York Style cheesecake with black cherry swirl (150 cal., 5 g. fat)	Frozen Mixed Berry Swirl New York Style cheesecake (1/8 pie=340 cal., 19 g. fat)

Sweet tooth selections (cont.)

Choose...	Instead Of...
One-crust pies (pumpkin, fruit tarts) (1/12 of Sara Lee Pumpkin pie =173 cal., 7 g. fat)	Two-crust fruit pies (1/12 pie=330 cal., 15 g. fat)
Mini scoop of key lime pie sherbet (1/4 cup=60 cal., 1 g. fat)	A slice of key lime pie (400 cal., 26 g. fat)
Mini scoop of raspberry sorbet (Haagen Dazs brand) (1/4 cup=55 cal., 0 g. fat)	1/2 cup of gourmet raspberry truffle ice cream (or similar) (290 cal., 20 g. fat)
1/2 cup strawberry or lemon yogurt blended with 1/2 cup fruit and 1/4 cup "light" Cool Whip (180 cal., 4 g. fat, plus 1.5 g. fiber)	1 thin slice of lemon or strawberry mousse cake (260 cal., 14 g. fat)

11 sugar surprises

Be careful with those fat-free and non-fat food products. If they have less fat than the original version but almost as many calories...that's your first clue that the sugar level may be through the roof. Check the label to be sure. These are the sugar surprises I found while hunting around my supermarket:

1. Sweetened tea and coffee drinks
(8 oz., 120 cal., 6 tsp. added sugar)

These fancy drinks have six or more teaspoons of sugar per one-cup serving! Try to find an unsweetened or artificially sweetened iced tea you care for.

2. Flavored instant oatmeal
(1 packet, 150 cal., 3 1/2 tsp. added sugar)

These convenient hot cereal products contain around four teaspoons of sugar per packet! Try making the plain unflavored packet of instant oatmeal and add one teaspoon of brown sugar or maple syrup.

3. Cottage cheese w/ strawberry sauce
(5.5 oz., 140 cal., 3 3/4 tsp. added sugar)

Try regular cottage cheese blended with fresh sliced strawberries.

4. Cherry flavored yogurt
(8 oz., 220 cal., 8 1/2 tsp. added sugar)

Try the light version of the same flavor yogurt.

5. Lemonade
(8 oz., 110 cal., 7 tsp. added sugar)

Try "light" lemonade (with artificial sweeteners) or make a blend of half real lemonade and half "light."

6. Frosted Strawberry Pop Tarts
(1 oz., 200 cal., 4 3/4 tsp. added sugar)

Try a piece of whole wheat toast with two teaspoons of strawberry jam.

7. Pancake syrup
(1/4 cup, 210 cal., 10 tsp. added sugar)

Try "light" reduced calorie pancake syrup.

8. Cinnamon applesauce
(4 oz., 100 cal., 6 tsp. added sugar)

Try unsweetened applesauce with a sprinkle of cinnamon.

9. Fruit cocktail canned in syrup
(1/2 cup, 100 cal., 5 3/4 tsp. added sugar)

Try "light" chunky mixed fruit.

10. Blueberry muffin (packed)
(1 muffin [4 oz.], 420 cal., 8 1/2 tsp. added sugar)

Try two Eggo frozen blueberry waffles.

11. Bottled flavored cold coffee drinks
(9.5 oz., 190 cal., 7 1/2 tsp. added sugar)

Try cooled brewed coffee with two tablespoons flavored non-dairy creamer.

Look to the nutrition label

When it comes to sugar, almost all processed and packaged products are suspect. Read the labels. I usually look at both the ingredient list and the nutrition label. Between the two of them I get a good idea of whether a product is high in added sugar. The Nutrition Facts label generally lists the total amount of carbohydrate and the grams of sugar per serving. Definitely look at the label to get an idea of whether that food product is higher in sugar than you would like it to be.

Definitions:

- **Total carbohydrate** = how many grams of total carbohydrate (sugars and starches) you get in a serving of food (calculated as the difference remaining after measuring its amount of protein, fat, ash, and moisture).
- **Sugars** = includes the total amount of sugars per serving—counting both added and natural sugars in the food. The grams of sugars are included in the total of carbohydrate listed on the label.
- **Sweeteners** = this term includes all types of sugar (raw, brown, powdered, granulated), honey, corn syrup, high fructose corn syrup, invert sugar, maple syrup, and fruit juice concentrates.

Shopping for less fat

Remember which foods contribute the most fat in the American diet? (If you need to refresh your memory, turn to Chapter 4.) Looking at this list, one of the simplest ways to skim the extra fat from these foods is to:

1. Buy the leaner cuts of beef and pork.
   Beef:
   - Eye of round (roast or steak).
   - Round tip (kebab).
   - Top loin (New York, club, or strip steak).

- Tenderloin (filet mignon, filet steak).
- Sirloin (sirloin steak, London broil).
- Top round.

(All have 8 grams of fat or less and 80 milligrams of cholesterol or less per 3-ounce portion, cooked and trimmed.)

Pork:
- Tenderloin with 4 grams fat and 67 milligrams cholesterol per 3-ounce cooked portion.
- Boneless sirloin chops.
- Boneless loin roasts.
- Top loin chops.
- Center loin chops.
- Sirloin roasts, boneless rib roasts and rib chops have 175 to 179 calories, 8.5 to 8.8 grams fat and 69 to 73 milligrams of cholesterol per 3-ounce lean, cooked portion.

2. Eat smaller portions when we have it.
3. Eat red meat less often and cook it without a lot of added fat.
4. Cut down on our use of margarine when we can.
5. Choose salad dressings that are not too high in fat and use canola oil or olive oil (see list below). You can also make a tasty mayonnaise blend by mixing 1/3 real mayonnaise and 2/3 cup fat-free or "light" sour cream. Some canola oil mayonnaise brands are also available.
6. Buy the better tasting reduced-fat cheeses. Use less cheese in recipes that seem to call for more cheese than necessary.
7. Buy lower-fat milks for cooking and drinking when possible. Whole milk can be used in place of cream in some recipes.
8. Follow guidelines in Chapter 4 for baking cakes, cookies, and quick breads with less fat than the original recipe.
9. Enjoy poultry without the skin when possible. Try to cook your chicken without a lot of added fat.

Shopping for salad dressings and spreads

	Cal.	Carb. (g)	Fat (g)
Mayonnaise: 1 tablespoon[1]			
Safeway Select Real Mayonnaise w/ canola	100	0	11
Spectrum Canola Mayo	100	0	12
Spectrum Lite Canola Eggless Mayonnaise	35	1	3
Salad dressing: 2 tablespoons[2]			
Kraft Special Collection			
Sun Dried Tomato	60	4	4.5
Italian Pesto	70	5	0.5
Balsamic Vinaigrette	110	1	12
Kraft—Light Done Right			
Red Wine Vinaigrette	50	3	4.5
Italian	50	2	4.5
Raspberry Vinaigrette	60	6	4
Cucumber Ranch	60	2	5.5
Catalina	80	9	5
Kraft			
Roasted Garlic Vinaigrette	50	3	4.5
Caesar Parmesan	60	1	5
Newman's Own			
Dynamite Lite Italian	45	3	4
Balsamic Vinaigrette	90	3	9

[1]Mayonnaise: 80 mg. sodium or less and 1 g. saturated fat per serving.
[2]Salad dressing: Between 230 and 480 mg. sodium and 1 g. saturated fat per serving.

10. Use less cooking oil in baking and cooking whenever possible. Switch to canola oil or olive oil in recipes depending on the recipe.

11. Use less other fat in baking and cooking whenever possible and switch to canola or olive oil in recipes whenever possible.

12. Check labels to find information on the yeast breads you like.

13. Enjoy potato chips and popcorn occasionally. Buy the reduced fat versions if you have tried them and enjoy them.

14. Buy reduced-fat or "light" sausage when possible—hopefully you will find a brand that you like.

15. An egg or two in bakery-type recipes is fine. But in most egg dishes, you can use half eggs and half egg whites or egg substitute and it should turn out very well.

16. Although nuts and seeds contribute some fat, they also contain vitamins, minerals, fiber, and phytochemicals. But certainly eating big spoon of peanut butter out of the jar fresh from the fridge is going to add up quickly. Try spreading peanut butter lightly on whole grains when possible. And when snacking on peanuts or sun-flower seeds, keep it to a handful or two instead of a bowlful.

17. Sometimes butter is the right fat for the particular recipe. In these cases, use butter, but just use less of it. If you can, replace it in that particular recipe with canola or olive oil.

When a frozen entrée is in order

I have found there are two types of people—people who seek out frozen entrées, and people who avoid them like the plague. However, frozen entrées can come in handy in many situations—as a quick lunch during the work week and as an easy dinner if you live alone or with one other person. I usually have a frozen pizza on hand in case of a meal emergency. (I've included frozen pizza information too.)

The problem with frozen entrées is this: The ones that are lower in fat are almost always too low in calories and carbohydrates.

Frozen entrées

	Cal.	Fat (g) (%[1])	Fib. (g)	Sat. fat(g)	Sod. (mg)
Frozen pizza					
DiGiorno Four Cheese Pizza (1/3 of a 12 oz. pizza)	280	9(29%)	2	5	700
Wolfgang Puck's Mushroom & Spinach Pizza (1/2 of a 10.5 oz. pizza)	270	8(27%)	5[2]	3	380
Wolfgang Puck's Four Cheese Pizza, (1/2 of a 9.25 oz. pizza)	360	15(37%)	5	6	530
Three-Cheese Oreida Bagel Bites (4 pieces)	190	6(28%)	1	3.5	530
Healthy Choice					
Chicken Enchiladas Suiza	280	6(19%)	5	3	440
Shrimp & Vegetables	270	6(20%)	6	3	580
Herb Baked Fish	340	7(19%)	5	1.5	480
Traditional Breast of Turkey	290	4.5(14%)	5	2	460
Chicken Enchilada Suprema	300	7(21%)	4	3	560
Lean Cuisine					
Chicken w/ Basil Cream Sauce	270	7(23%)	3	2	580
Chicken in Peanut Sauce	290	6(19%)	4	1.5	590
Baked Fish w/ Cheddar Shells	270	6(20%)	4	2	540
Fiesta Chicken (with black beans, rice, and vegetables)	270	5(17%)	4.5	5	90
Cheese Lasagna w/ Lightly Breaded Chicken Breast Scallopini	290	8(25%)	3	2	590
Shrimp & Angel Hair Pasta	290	6(19%)	1	1	590
3-Bean Chili	250	6(22%)	9	2	590
The Budget Gourmet					
Three Cheese Lasagna	310	12(35%)	2	6	700
Fettucini and Meatballs in Wine Sauce w/ Green Beans	270	7(23%)	3	3	560

Frozen entrées (cont.)

	Cal.	Fat (g) (%[1])	Fib. (g)	Sat. fat(g)	Sod. (mg)
Marie Calender's					
Chili & Cornbread	540	21(35%)	**7**	9	2,110
Sweet & Sour Chicken	570	15(24%)	**7**	2.5	700
Beef Tips in Mushroom Sauce	430	17(36%)	6	7	1,620
Turkey w/ Gravy and Dressing	500	19(34%)	4	9	2,040
Spaghetti and Meat Sauce	670	25(34%)	**9**	11	1,160
Stuffed Pasta Trio	640	18(25%)	**5**	9	950
Swanson					
Mexican Style Combination	470	18(34%)	**5**	6	1,610
Chicken Parmigiana	370	17(41%)	4	5	1,010
Herb Roasted Chicken Breast Tenders w/ Rice & Vegetables	310	7(20%)	3	2.5	780
Turkey Dinner	310	8.5(25%)	**5**	2	890

[1]Percent of calories from fat.
[2]Bold type denotes that fiber content equals five grams or higher.

They are meager in the vegetable department. Many contain around 300 calories—the number of calories in one measly bagel. In order to make the entrées more nutritious and satisfying you might consider adding fruits and vegetables. You might even need to add some cooked rice, noodles, or even some grated cheese.

Some frozen entrées are brimming with sodium, and others aren't that bad (check the table and you'll see what I mean). If you need to watch your sodium intake, keep an eye on this portion of the nutrition label.

Shopping for antioxidants

Remember the antioxidants in Chapters 2 through 4? They work by neutralizing highly reactive, destructive compounds called free radicals. The best places to go for antioxidants are the fruit, vegetable, and whole grain sections of your supermarket (foods provide better insurance than do supplements that you're getting the antioxidants in the right amount and form and in the right combinations.) Here are some of the best supermarket sources of the four most studied antioxidants.

Vitamin C

The body cannot store this powerful antioxidant, so we need to get some of it every day.

- Citrus fruits.
- Green peppers.
- Broccoli.
- Green leafy vegetables.

- Strawberries.
- Raw cabbage.
- Potatoes.

Vitamin E

A fat-soluble vitamin, that can be stored with fat in the liver and other tissues. This powerful antioxidant can be found in a range of plant foods, such as:

- Wheat germ.
- Nuts.
- Seeds.

- Whole grains.
- Green leafy vegetables.
- Vegetable oil.

Beta-carotene

This is one of the 600 different carotenoids that have been discovered, by far the most studied of the 600. Beta carotene protects dark green, yellow and orange vegetables and fruits from solar radiation damage. So that's where you'll find it!

- Carrots.
- Squash.
- Broccoli.
- Sweet potatoes.
- Tomatoes.

- Kale.
- Collards.
- Cantaloupe.
- Peaches.
- Apricots.

Selenium

This is a mineral antioxidant that is thought to help fight cell damage and may help protect against cancer. Because it is a mineral, amounts can accumulate in the body. Large doses of the supplement form of selenium, for example, can be toxic. It is best to get selenium through the following foods.

- Fish.
- Shellfish.
- Red meat.
- Grains.
- Eggs.

- Chicken.
- Garlic.
- Vegetables grown in selenium-rich soils.

Frozen foods—for winter relief

How do you get the antioxidant vitamins A and C in the dead of winter when fresh produce is scarce? Find your frozen food section of your supermarket. Frozen foods have an advantage over canned when it comes to water-soluble vitamin C and beta-carotene. Water-soluble vitamins leach into water during the canning and cooking process. When flash freezing fruits and vegetables, much of the nutrients are preserved well. But to keep the antioxidant levels high:

- Don't overheat your frozen vegetables (cook just until tender).
- Use only a minimum of water when cooking.
- Microwaving or steaming are your best choices.

You'll find ample carotene (Vitamin A) in:

- Frozen carrots (1295 RE per 1/2 cup).
- Frozen peas and carrots (625 RE per 1/2 cup).
- Frozen spinach (875 RE per 1/2 cup).
- Frozen kale (475 per 1/2 cup).

You'll find ample vitamin C in:

- Orange juice concentrate.
- Frozen, unsweetened strawberries.
- Broccoli spears.
- Vegetable medleys with red and green peppers.
- Vegetable medleys with broccoli florets.

- Grape juice from concentrate (60 mg. per cup) when vitamin C is added in processing (check label).
- Frozen sliced peaches (235 mg. per cup) when vitamin C is added in processing (check label).

Shopping for cabbage family vegetables

Here are the members of the cabbage family and some helpful hints on how to buy, store, and use them.

Brussels sprouts
- Available year round frozen, but best between October and March.
- When picking them out look for firm, compact, sprouts with a good green color.
- Serving suggestions: Boiled and steamed, often served with sauces or butter.

Cauliflower
- Available year round, but generally heavier in September, October, and November.
- When picking them out the head should be white or slightly creamy white, very firm and compact.
- Serving suggestions: Avoid overcooking (whether steaming or in the microwave). When the stem end yields to the touch of the fork, boiled cauliflower is done.

Cabbage
- Available year round.
- When picking them out look for solid heads, heavy for the size and showing no discolored veins.
- Serving suggestions: Add to slow cooker in last 60 minutes of cooking, add to stir fry toward the end of cooking, microwave or steam too.

Broccoli
- Available year round. A small supply is available in July and August.
- When picking them out look for green color in the heads as well as the leaves and stems. Stalks should be

tender and firm with compact dark green or purplish-green buds in the head.
- Serving suggestions: Use as little water as possible when cooking and use rapid cooking like microwave, steaming, or stir frying.

Mustard greens
- Available year round.
- When picking them out they should be tender, and crisp, and of good, green color.
- Serving suggestions: the young tender leaves can be used as salad leaves, either alone or mixed with other salad greens. Older, tender leaves are used for cooking.

Kale
(A large, curly-leafed green)
- Available throughout winter.
- When picking them out look for dark green leaves that are crisp, clean, and free from bruising and crushing.
- Serving suggestions: cut off and discard root ends, tough stems, and discolored leaves. Cut off and discard midribs. Wash, lift out of water, and shake leaves well. Serve raw or cooked (cook like other greens).

Kohlrabi
(Has a delicate turnip-like flavor and looks a little like celery, but with thinner ribs and a bulb-shaped bottom. (Bulb, stems, and leaves are all good to eat.)
- Available June through October.
- When picking them out choose young, tender bulbs with fresh, green leaves; avoid those with scars and blemishes. The smaller the bulb the more delicate the flavor and texture.
- Serving suggestions: Boil, steam, or microwave. Scrub well and peel if bulbs are to be sliced or diced before cooking. Serve sliced small raw kohlrabi with a dip for an appetizer. Add diced raw kohlrabi to stews and soups during the last 20 minutes of cooking. Stir-fry with other vegetables.

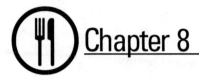 Chapter 8

Restaurant Rules

Nowadays, many of us now eat out more than we eat in. We have busy lifestyles and eating out just becomes part of the "working and on the go" equation. We can't help it! Or can we?

Busy American families can definitely make more of an effort to cook at home. Sometimes it seems like nobody is cooking anymore (more on this in Chapter 6). However, we can do a better job of eating healthy when we eat out, especially because many of us eat out almost every day. In general, foods selected and eaten away from home are slightly higher in fat and cholesterol, and slightly lower in other nutrients compared to foods eaten at home. This probably doesn't surprise you.

Where is America eating out?

Of people who ate out in 1994 and 1995 and were part of the 1994-96 Continuing Survey of Food Intakes conducted by the USDA Food Surveys Research Group:

- 33 percent chose a fast food place (which includes pizza parlors).
- 27 percent chose a restaurant with table service.
- 25 percent bought and ate food from a grocery or convenience store.

Which meals do Americans eat out?

Lunch or brunch is the most common meal eaten out. Snacks or beverage breaks come in second, and about 25 percent of us are eating breakfast away from home.

It's all about choices. We have lots of choices out there in restaurant and fast food land. We choose where we go, what we order, and how much we eat when we eat out. This chapter will help you figure out the first two choices, so that you are actually following some of those 10 food steps to freedom, even when you are eating out.

Food Step 1: Eat 5 to 10 servings of fruits and vegetables a day

Believe it or not, ordering vegetables when eating in restaurants is a natural thing to do. Restaurants do such as great job of preparing and presenting food, and vegetables are no exception. It's a delight to eat vegetables—at least that's been my experience.

- Order a green or spinach salad with dressing on the side.
- When they give you a choice of side dishes, choose the sides that include vegetables.
- Many restaurants garnish the plate with some fresh fruit. Go ahead and eat that wedge of cantaloupe, pineapple, or slice of orange. If there is no fruit to be found on the plate (or on the menu), ask if they have fresh fruit.
- Look for fruit salad selections in delis and restaurants.
- If there is a vegetable entrée you think sounds interesting, you might want to give it try—instead of the meat and potato plan.

Food Step 2: Eat cabbage family vegetables several times a week

- Broccoli is often the seasonal vegetable served on the side of your entrée. If so, enjoy! You've just eaten a member of the cabbage family.
- There's more to the cabbage family than broccoli, so keep your eyes peeled looking for any of the other members to be offered on the menu.

- If you are at a salad bar, grab some extra broccoli and cauliflower for your salad. All you need is 1/2 cup (about a scoop) to equal a serving of cabbage family vegetables.

Food Step 3: Eat omega-3 rich fish several times a week

- Eating at a nice restaurant is a fabulous time to have your fish. I try to order items in restaurants that I don't normally have at home—which, for me, is shellfish. Although I eat salmon and other fish fillets quite often at home, it's also fun for me to try the creative ways that restaurants prepare it.
- Albacore tuna salad sandwiches count as a fish serving with omega-3s. So if you are at a deli and the albacore tuna sandwich looks good, go for it.
- Some ethnic restaurants offer great fish entrees, such as salmon teriyaki at a Japanese restaurant, fish tacos at Mexican restaurants, and shrimp at Chinese restaurants.

Food Step 4: Eat less red meat (and more beans)

- This is going to be a tough one for people who love to eat beef or pork when they go to a restaurant. When you can, try something that is more along the line of chicken or fish.
- Many ethnic restaurants offer a tasty way to squeeze beans into a dish. Mexican restaurants offer beans on the side or you can order your burrito with beans instead of beef. You might see beans on the menu in Indian and Mediterranean restaurants as well.
- You can even find beans at fast food Mexican restaurants. Bean burritos or ordering a side of beans is a good way to go.
- Some delis or sandwich shops offer three-bean salads dressed in vinaigrette.

Food Step 5: Eat less saturated fat and avoid eating a high-fat diet

- Trying to eat less meat, and eat more fish, when eating out will help accomplish this food step.

- We tend to eat higher-fat meals when we eat out, so this food step is probably the hardest to follow. One of the simplest ways to eat less fat when eating out is to avoid deep fried items. That's tough in fast food restaurants, but it can be done.

Food Step 6: Keep extra weight off

- One of our biggest mistakes when eating out is that we eat too much. We are enjoying the meal and the company, and perhaps we push ourselves to clean our plate.
- Resist the urge to join the clean plate club. Slow down, drink water between bites, pace yourself. If you listen when your stomach tells you it is comfortable, you'll probably end up with food left on your plate.
- Anticipate eating leftovers later that day, or the next.

Food Step 7: Eat several servings of whole grains a day

- It's difficult to find whole grains at restaurants and fast food places. Some might offer whole grain breads, or your chicken sandwich might be served on a multigrain bun.
- Some Chinese restaurants offer the option of steamed brown rice.
- Look for barley soup, or other dishes with barley, on the menu.
- On the days that you eat out and can't get a serving of whole grain in, enjoy a whole grain cereal earlier, or later, in the day as a snack.

Food Step 8: Consider taking a multivitamin containing some folate, calcium, and vitamin E

- Take your multivitamin as normally scheduled. Some people take it with a particular meal. Others get to it at the end of the day when they are brushing their teeth.

Food Step 9: Don't overdo sugary foods and alcohol (and drink more than 5 glasses of plain water every day)

- Enjoy the glass of ice water that restaurants set down on the table when you arrive. It will help you quench your thirst without turning to drinks with alcohol or sugar.
- Restaurants have the most fabulous desserts! If you can talk your table guests into it, it's fun to decide on one of the desserts, and let everyone at the table taste it.
- Soda is one of the biggest contributors of added sugar in the American diet. There are lots of other options at most restaurants. Iced tea is a nice change from soda and most fast food places have it. Fast food chains will gladly give you a cup of ice water—all you have to do is ask.

Food Step 10: Stay active and exercise as much as possible

- After a restaurant meal, take a 10-minute walk if you can. Stretch your legs and get your body moving. You'll be a lot more comfortable afterwards and you'll have added 10 minutes of exercise to your day.

Eating out = 300 extra calories and 20 more grams of fat

How many times did you eat out or order in last week, including those quick breakfast stops and deli lunches? If you're like most Americans, the answer is at least four times. In fact, the number of people eating fast food has doubled in the past decade.

A recent study in the *Journal of the American Dietetic Association* found that women who eat out more than five times a week consume almost 300 more calories and nearly 20 more grams of fat per day than those who eat most meals at home. About 38 percent of calories in the average restaurant meal come from fat. All of this doesn't exactly help with maintaining a healthy weight. In fact, it may be sabotaging you.

The advice below is broken down into fast food and/or restaurant tips. Some of us have a tendency toward one or the other. But let's face it, most of us frequent both on a regular basis. In my house, we are thrilled to get a chance to go to a restaurant (most of our meals are homemade). We keep our fast food visits to once a week. I think back to when I was a child. Only if it was somebody's birthday, would we get to go to McDonald's—it was a big deal for us to go to any kind of restaurant. Times have definitely changed in the last 30 years. Not all of it is bad, but it all comes back around to making better choices.

Have your fast food and eat it too
(includes pizza, delis, and bagel shops)

Fast food has a bad reputation when it comes to eating healthy. On the positive side, some of the chains have made some lower fat items available, such as grilled chicken sandwiches or rice bowls. You will still be hard pressed to find a whole serving of fruits, vegetables, or whole grains anywhere, though.

1. The pita sandwiches at Wendy's can be made with reduced-fat Caesar vinaigrette, (70 calories, 7 grams fat per tablespoon) or reduced-fat garden ranch sauce (50 calories, 4.5 grams fat per tablespoon). Choose from Chicken Caesar Pita or two vegetarian choices; Garden Veggie and Classic Greek Pita.

2. Many fast food chains now offer grilled chicken sandwiches. Have one with a side salad (dressed with reduced calorie ranch dressing, for example). Compared to a chicken club sandwich and small fries, you'll cut over 300 calories and half the fat.

3. Fast food chains do sell fish; that's the good news. The bad news is, they deep-fry it. If you eat your fish sandwich without tartar sauce (or at least scrape off most of it) you make it a much better bet.

4. If you've just got to have that burger, make sure it's no larger than a quarter-pound. Pass up the high-fat toppings (bacon, cheese, mayonnaise, or special sauce) for the lighter options (mustard, catsup, barbecue sauce, lettuce, onion, tomato, and hot peppers). The

smallest hamburgers (the size that come in the kid meals) are you absolute best bets, because they have the least amount of burger per square inch of bun, and are usually made without mayonnaise or other creamy sauces.

5. Some fast foods offer baked potato meals that are worth biting into. They do a great job providing you up with at least 8 grams of fiber.

6. Downsize your meat order and stop ordering large fries. A double or 1/2-pound burger with mayonnaise or special sauce has more than twice the calories, and nearly four times the fat, of a regular 1/4-pound burger dressed with ketchup, BBQ sauce, or mustard. A small order of fries saves you around 200 calories and 10 grams of fat.

7. Pass up the "supreme" or "deluxe" sized item in favor of the regular version at any fast food restaurant. At the Taco Bell fast food chain, for example, a soft taco made with grilled meat contains half the fat and one-third fewer calories than a "taco supreme." And a "big beef burrito" has over 20 percent fewer calories and over 25 percent less fat than the "big beef burrito supreme."

Pizza tips

8. Hold the toppings on your pizza. Leave the pepperoni, sausage, and extra cheese off a thin-crust pizza, and it becomes a healthy dish that gets around 30 percent of its calories from fat.

9. Top your pizza with your favorite veggies to you'll boost the fiber and vitamin totals all at the same time. A 1/4 cup each of green peppers, onions, and mushrooms adds just 26 calories, along with 1.5 grams fiber, 26 milligrams vitamin C, 9 percent of the RDA of folic acid, and 8 percent of the RDA for vitamins B2, B3, and B6.

10. Stick to two large slices of pizza in one sitting. If you are still hungry, have some fruit, a bowl of soup, or a green salad.

11. The more authentic your pizza (when the pizza is made with a better bread crust and light on the cheese), the lower in fat the crust will be.

12. Condiments do count. Choose catsup, mustard, or BBQ sauce for your fish or chicken sandwich (instead of mayonnaise, special sauce, or tartar sauce) and it will have 100 to 200 fewer calories and 10 to 20 grams less fat. Ask for Bull's Eye Barbecue Sauce on your Whopper sandwich instead of the usual mayonnaise, and you'll cut calories by 20 percent, and fat grams by over 40 percent.

13. Bread is best for breakfast sandwiches and stay away from sausage (if you can help it). Just ordering your breakfast sandwich on a bagel or English muffin instead of a higher fat and calorie biscuit or croissant will trim off over 100 calories and 10 grams of fat. An Egg McMuffin from McDonald's, for example, is certainly a better bet with 290 calories and 12 grams of fat than a sausage biscuit with 470 calories and 31 grams of fat.

14. Buy beans when you can. Beans are filled with fiber, phytochemicals, vitamins, and minerals. Some fast food chains offer entrees or side dishes containing beans—like the bean burrito from Taco Bell (12 grams of fiber, 370 calories, and 12 of grams fat), or the side of pintos 'n cheese (10 grams of fiber, 180 calories, and 8 grams of fat). Wendy's offers a small cup of chili with 5 grams of fiber, 210 calories, and 7 grams of fat.

15. B.Y.O.P. (Bring Your Own Produce). Getting fruits and vegetables at almost every meal is one of the best health steps we can take. It's no surprise that fast food is sorely lacking in the produce department (French fries don't really count). Make a habit to bring you own. Chew on carrots and apple slices on your way there. Not only will it head off your hunger—it will bring your daily fruit and vegetable count up by two servings!

16. Watch the beverages. When you are thirsty, your body wants water. And fast food chains are all happy to give you an ice water. Other good choices are reduced-fat milk (most chains have it now), orange juice, and iced tea (if a little bit of caffeine doesn't bother you). Go for a soda or shake and your meal jumps up 200 calories for a 16-ounce soda or about 350 calories for a small size shake (it also adds 7 to 9 grams to your fat total).

17. Ditch dessert. Not to say that dessert can't be enjoyed sometimes, but buying dessert each time you buy a fast food meal is an expensive habit to get into. A little apple pie from Burger King will cost you 300 calories and 15 grams of fat (or 260 calories and 13 grams of fat at McDonald's). And a small frosty from Wendy's will run you 330 calories and 8 grams of fat.

18. Grab a bagel with an ounce of light cream cheese from a bagel shop. And choose a whole grain or an oat bran bagel if they're available—the fiber you will get goes up to 5.5 and 8 grams, respectively.

Sandwich/deli tips

19. Request whole wheat bread, rolls, or bagels to pump up the nutrition in your sandwich.

20. Hold the mayo. Order your sandwich with catsup or mustard. Sometimes Italian delis will lightly wet the bread with an olive oil mixture, which at least adds the more desirable monounsaturated fat. If you must have mayonnaise, ask them to spread it very lightly.

21. Choose leaner meat fillings such as roast chicken, roast turkey, roast beef, or lean ham.

22. Order your sandwich with a fresh fruit (like an orange or apple) or a fruit salad.

23. Enjoy light versions of your favorite chicken, shrimp, and tuna salad sandwiches at home.

Today's best drive-through dinners

Should you find yourself in a fast food drive through, and you just want to know what your best choices are, I've listed some below. After all, this book is titled "Tell Me What to Eat..."

- Chicken Teriyaki Bowl (Jack in the Box) contains 670 calories, 4 g. fat (5 percent calories from fat), 3 g. fiber, (this is high in sodium though—1730 mg.).
- Grilled Chicken sandwich (Wendy's) contains 310 calories, 8 g. fat (23 percent calories from fat), 2 g. fiber.
- The BK Broiler Chicken sandwich (without mayonnaise) (Burger King) totals 370 calories, 9 g. fat (22 percent calories from fat), 2 g. fiber.
- Fish Sandwich without tartar sauce (Burger King) contains 460 calories, 14 g. fat (27 percent calories from fat), 3 g. fiber.
- Filet-O-Fish without tartar sauce (McDonald's) contains 398 calories, 12 g. fat (27 percent calories from fat), 2 g. fiber.
- Chicken Caesar Pita (Wendy's) contains 490 calories, 18 g. fat (33 percent calories from fat), 4 g. fiber.
- Garden Veggie Pita (Wendy's) contains 400 calories, 17 g. fat (38 percent calories from fat), 5 g. fiber.
- Sour Cream and Chives potato (Wendy's) contains 380 calories, 6 g. fat (14 percent calories from fat), 8 g. fiber.
- Broccoli & Cheese Potato (Wendy's) contains 470 calories, 14 g. fat (27 percent calories from fat), 9 g. fiber.
- Chicken Fajita Pita (Jack in the Box) contains 280 calories, 9 g. fat (29 percent calories from fat), 3 g. fiber.
- BBQ Flavored Chicken sandwich (Kentucky Fried Chicken) contains 356 calories, 8 g. fat (28 percent calories from fat), 2 g. fiber.
- The Hamburger (smallest) (McDonald's) contains 250 calories, 9 g. fat (32 percent Calories from fat), 2 g. fiber.
- The Jr. Hamburger (Wendy's) contains 270 calories, 10 g. fat (33 percent calories from fat), 2 g. fiber.

- Whopper Jr. (without mayonnaise) (Burger King) contains 320 calories, 15 g. fat (42 percent calories from fat), 2 g. fiber.
- Grilled Chicken Salad (McDonald's) made with half a package of Caesar dressing totals 200 calories, 8.5 g. fat (38 percent calories from fat), 3 g. fiber.
- Grilled Steak or Chicken Soft Tacos (Taco Bell) contains 200 calories, 7 g. fat (31 percent Calories from fat), 2 g. fiber each.
- Bean Burrito (Taco Bell) contains 370 calories, 12 g. fat (29 percent calories from fat), 12 g. fiber.
- Grilled Chicken Burrito (Taco Bell) contains 390 calories, 13 g. fat (30 percent calories from fat), 3 g. fiber.

30 ways you can eat right when eating at restaurants

For most of us, eating out or ordering in means eating more calories than we would otherwise. But remember you do have options...

Breakfast and diner tips

1. If you often order a 3-egg omelet at your favorite breakfast, ask them to use egg substitute and choose the ham, cheese, and vegetable filling instead of the sausage and cheese filling. (This will cut over 350 calories, 600 milligrams of cholesterol, and 3/4 of the fat.)

2. Instead of having your breakfast with two sausage links, ask for a large grilled slice of ham instead. (You'll cut over 150 calories and 15 grams of fat).

3. Skillet potatoes, made with chunks of potato, should (depending on the restaurant) be a little less greasy than hash browns. You can always request that the potatoes be made with a minimum of oil.

4. A plate of buttermilk pancakes with a strip or two of bacon shouldn't get you into too much trouble, as long as you go light on the butter.

5. If you are choosing between a couple of strips of bacon or two links of sausage, go for the bacon. Even though we think of bacon as fatty, a typical side order of sausage contains even more fat.

6. If you like to order deep-fried or sautéed shellfish dishes when you eat out, you can start ordering grilled seafood instead, to cut extra calories. (You'll cut about 150 calories and 2/3 of the fat.)
7. If you like ordering a beef burrito at Mexican restaurants, enjoy a bean burrito without some of the extras instead. (You'll cut about 150 calories and half the fat.) Or enjoy a grilled chicken burrito.
8. If you have a hankering for a cheeseburger and fries meal, have oven fries some other time at home (this might be asking too much), and go for the smallest burger on the menu (like a 1/4 pounder instead of a 1/3 or 1/2 pound hamburger). You can dress it with catsup and mustard instead of high calorie "special sauce" and mayonnaise.
9. Enjoy ethnic foods, such as Indian and Asian, that are naturally light or vegetarian.

The rotisserie and other restaurants

10. Order a roasted chicken breast and baked potato with a spoon of sour cream instead of a chicken pot pie. (This will cut about 500 calories and 2/3 of the fat of the pot pie.)
11. Enjoy sliced turkey breast or lean ham with new potatoes, steamed vegetables, and hot cinnamon apples. This will amount to about 595 calories, with 9 grams of fat (only 2 grams saturated fat).
12. Opt for the roasted chicken, and skip the skin (that's where most of the fat is). If you must have some, eat a few bites of the crispy bits you can't resist, and toss the rest.
13. Pass up such creamy side dishes as creamed spinach and ask for the baked new potatoes, sweet potatoes, zucchini marinara, rice pilaf, red beans, rice, steamed vegetables, or fresh fruit.
14. The meatloaf sandwich (without cheese) should keep your fat in check, especially if you have it with low fat vegetable soup and/or fruits and vegetables.

15. Chicken noodle soup (and most other clear soups) with corn bread can make a nice light lunch or dinner.

16. At an Italian restaurant, order pasta with meat sauce or meat tortellini with marinara, instead of higher fat pastas such as fettuccine Alfredo or pasta carbonara. (You'll cut the fat in half.)

17. High-fat, buttery, or creamy sauces should be garnishes, not large portions of the meal. Ask for half as much of these sauces when ordering pasta or meat dishes.

18. Ask to substitute marinara, marsala, or wine sauces for cream and butter sauces that come with chicken, fish, or pasta.

19. When at Chinese restaurants, order the stir-fried dishes made with lean meat, fish, and lots of vegetables and try not to order too many of those deep fried dishes and appetizers.

20. Go for grilled or roasted chicken pieces, or a grilled chicken sandwich and forget the fried chicken dinner or the breaded and fried chicken sandwich. You will be rewarded with 150 fewer calories and half the fat. Ordering the 1/4 roasted chicken (white meat, no skin) at Boston Market, for example, buys you just 170 calories, 4 grams of fat, and a whopping 33 grams of protein (not including side dishes).

21. Ask for salad dressing on the side. This way you decide how much you add to your salad.

22. Some of our favorite comfort foods, like pot roast or turkey dinners, are actually some of the lowest fat entrees at home-style restaurants.

23. Grilled fish is a great dinner choice. Not only does fish contain beneficial omega-3 fatty acids, but it is also the type of dinner we tend not to make for ourselves at home.

24. At Chinese restaurants, you can ask that your stir-fried dishes be prepared with only a little oil. I've found most will oblige—all you have to do is ask. Even fried rice can be made with less oil. While you're at it, you

can also ask that the flavor-enhancing MSG be left out if it bothers you.

25. Try to reduce deep fried items at Chinese restaurants to appetizer-size portions instead of entrée size.

The steakhouse

26. Steakhouse servings are cowboy sized. Look forward to taking home half your meal for a great lunch tomorrow. Or order the "petite" or "junior" portions of meat when available.

27. If you tend to enjoy a T-bone steak when you eat out, try a leaner steak like filet mignon or sirloin, and trim off all the visible fat regardless of which cut you choose. (You'll cut about 200 calories and over half the fat). The fatter cuts are: rib eye, prime rib, porterhouse, and T-bone.

28. Enjoy a sirloin steak with BBQ dipping sauce instead of ribs. (You save about 250 calories and 2/3 of the fat.)

29. Have your meat dish with lots of vegetables that you like (beans may even be available). The vegetables will help fill you up so that you won't be tempted to overdo the meat. The vegetables and beans help boost nutrition and fiber totals too.

30. Eat side dishes that you enjoy, and that are lower in fat, to help balance out the beef. These might include a clear broth or tomato-based soup, baked potato (modest on butter and sour cream) or mashed potatoes, broccoli, beans, rice pilaf, dinner roll, cornbread, and cinnamon apples.

Chez moi

Going to restaurants is one of my favorite things! What's not to like? But if you are the least bit interested in enjoying light versions of recipes from famous restaurants across the country, you might be interested in one of my cookbooks, *Chez Moi: Lightening Up Famous Restaurant Recipes*. It's full of sought-after restaurant recipes that I've turned into reduced-fat treasures. Check it out at *www.amazon.com*, or on my Web site *www.recipedoctor.com*.

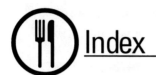 Index

A

alcohol, 146
  limiting, 77, 81-83
antioxidant recipes, 112-117
antioxidants, 21, 41-43,
  137-139
aspirin, 17-18

B

barium enema, 15
beans, 50-53, 144-145
  recipes with, 109-112
beta-carotene, 138
bile acids, 23
breads and bagels, 125, 126

C

cabbage family vegetables,
  143-144
  benefits of, 45-47
  shopping for, 140-141
  recipes with, 106-109
calcium, 28, 70, 72-74

calorie burning, maximizing
  your, 97-98
carbohydrates, 34-35
carcinogens, 22
  minimizing exposure to, 17
cereal, whole grain, 67-69,
  125, 127
colon cancer and connection
  to diet, 19-28
colon cancer facts, 5-6
colon cancer,
  defined, 7-8
  preventing, 17-18
  symptoms of, 11-12
colon, how it works, 24-26
colonoscopy, 5, 13-16
colorectal cancer, 16
colorectal tumors, 22-23
colorectal, 7
colostomy, 16-17

D

diabetes, type 2, 68
diet as a cancer risk, 29
diet and colon cancer, 19-28
digital rectal examination, 16

E

eating habits, 94-95
exercise, 33, 83-86, 146

F

fad diets, 33-34, 89, 92-93
fast food, 147-152
fat replacements, 60-61
fat sources, 55-57
fat,
    connection to colon cancer,
        27-28
    cooking with less, 58-59
    shopping for less, 132-135
    types of, 54-55
Fecal Occult Blood Testing
    (FOBT), 12-13
fiber and children, 31
fiber, 23-24, 26, 29-30, 44,
    64-66
fiber, connection to colon
    health 23-24
fish recipes, 117-121
fish, 32-33, 47-50, 144
flavonoids, 66
flaxseed, 32-33, 66
flexible sigmoidoscopy, 13, 15
folic acid, 44, 70-72
food and connection to cancer,
    39-88
food triggers, 96-97
free radicals, 21-22
frozen entrées, 135-137
frozen foods, 139-140
fruits and vegetables, 143
    importance of, 40-45
    recipes with, 112-117

G

garlic and cancer prevention,
    35-36
grains, whole, 63-70, 145
    recipes with, 102-105
grilling and connection to
    cancer, 31-32

H

heart disease, reducing the
    risk of, 68
heredity/genetics, as risk
    indicator, 10-11
hormone replacement therapy,
    17

I

iron, 50, 74

L

lignans, 66

M

motivation, finding source of,
    86-88
multivitamins, 70-77, 145

muscle mass, maintaining
   your, 98-100

N

nitrosamines, 32
nutrition labels,
   understanding, 132

O

omega-3 fatty acids, 27,
   32-33, 47-50, 144

P

pesticide residue and cancer
   connection, 36-37
phytochemicals, 41-43,
   45-46, 66-67
polyps, 7, 8
protein, 37-38

R

recipes, 101-121
red meat, 50-53, 144
research, future, 86
restaurant tips, 142-155
risk factors, 9-10

S

salad dressings and spreads,
   134

saturated fat, 53-53, 144-145
screening, 12, 14
selenium, 139
serum cholesterol, 68
sugar, 77-81, 126-131, 146
supermarket tips, 122-141
supplement, choosing a,
   74-77
symptoms of colon cancer,
   11-12

T

tocotrienols, 66

V

vitamin E, 70, 74
vitamins, 138

W

waffles, whole grain frozen,
   125-126, 128
water, 146
   importance of, 82-83
weight loss, quick, 90
weight vs. health, 89-100
weight, keeping off, 63, 145
whole grain products,
   124-128
whole grains, 63-70, 145
   recipes with, 102-105

LaVergne, TN USA
07 July 2010
188522LV00001B/43/A